Supporting Siblings
and Their Families
During Intensive Baby Care

Supporting Siblings and Their Families During Intensive Baby Care

by

Linda Rector

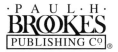

·P·A·U·L·H·
BROOKES
PUBLISHING CO®

Baltimore • London • Sydney

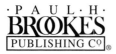

Paul H. Brookes Publishing Co.
Post Office Box 10624
Baltimore, Maryland 21285-0624

www.brookespublishing.com

Typeset by Graphic World, Inc., St. Louis, Missouri.
Manufactured in the United States of America by
Versa Press, Inc., East Peoria, Illinois.

Clinical vignettes are derived from the author's actual experiences. In all instances, pseudonyms have been used and identifying details have been changed to protect confidentiality.

Photographs on the front cover and on pages 29, 35, 37, 47, 55, 79, 87, 95, 105, 108, 115, and 141 courtesy of Texas Children's Hospital in Houston, Texas; Carol Turnage Carrier, photographer.

Photographs on pages 99 and 120 courtesy of Michelle Lawson.

Library of Congress Cataloging-in-Publication Data

Rector, Linda.
 Supporting siblings and their families during intensive baby care / by Linda Rector.
  p.   ; cm.
 Includes bibliographical references and index.
 ISBN-13: 978-1-55766-852-3 (pbk.)
 ISBN-10: 1-55766-852-3 (pbk.)
 1. Neonatal intensive care. 2. Premature infants—Hospital care—Social aspects.
 3. Medical social work. 4. Hospital patients—Family relationships. I. Title.
 [DNLM: 1. Sibling Relations. 2. Adaptation, Psychological. 3. Child Psychology.
 4. Infant, Newborn. 5. Intensive Care Units, Neonatal. 6. Siblings—psychology.
 7. Social Support. WS 105.5.F2 R311s 2007] I. Title.
 RJ253.5.R43 2007
 618.92'01—dc22   2006037293

British Library Cataloguing in Publication data are available from the British Library.

Contents

About the Author

Linda Rector, M.S., CCLS, Independent Consultant, Houston, Texas.

Ms. Rector is a Reach Out and Read Volunteer at the Good Neighbor Clinic in Houston, Texas. She served as a neonatal child life specialist for a number of years as well as a child life manager and child life specialist on a variety of units at Texas Children's Hospital in Houston, Texas. Ms. Rector also worked as a child life specialist at Driscoll Children's Hospital in Corpus Christi, Texas; a child life fellow at Children's Medical Center in Dallas, Texas; and a sixth-grade teacher at Calallen Independent School District in Corpus Christi, Texas.

Ms. Rector graduated from The Ohio State University with a master of science degree in child development and from Texas Christian University with a bachelor of science degree in elementary education. She is a certified child life specialist and is certified in Texas as an elementary teacher with a kindergarten endorsement.

In November 2001, Ms. Rector received the first annual Reba Michels Hill Award from Baylor College of Medicine, Department of Pediatrics, Section of Neonatology. In 1993, she was a member of the psychosocial team from Baylor College of Medicine, Houston VA Hospital, and Texas Children's Hospital requested to work with children released from Ranch Apocalypse (the Branch Davidians' compound) in Waco, Texas. She has given a number of presentations and interviews on topics such as the education, training, and role of neonatal child life specialists, infant brain development, pain management for infants, and debriefing protocols for traumatized children.

Foreword

It seems like only a few years ago when someone had the bright idea that family-centered care would help families develop ownership of their newborn in
the neonatal intensive care unit (NICU). As the idea gained momentum, the
"family" grew to include grandparents, aunts, uncles, identified support systems, and SIBLINGS. General panic broke out as staff expressed anxiety
about opening the doors of the NICU and letting children inside to create
chaos. Surprisingly enough, the concept caught on and is practiced in many
NICUs around the country. This book is long overdue as a resource for professionals and families dealing with siblings who have a brother or sister
needing NICU care. Linda Rector uses available research evidence and presents fictional case examples, supportive activities, and resources for working
with siblings of high-risk infants from the high-risk pregnancy, through hospitalization, and finally to adjustment to home life.

Throughout the book, short narratives describe sibling or family issues
or provide in story form ways to resolve difficult situations using simple
strategies. Ms. Rector uses these anecdotes to illustrate important points for
each chapter, leaving the reader with a practical message that can be used
to help families. Reading these stories, which go through each age group
and review ways in which children understand or cope with the pregnancy
or birth of a new brother or sister, is almost a virtual experience as the sim-
ulations stir the imagination back into childhood.

The importance of this book is that it demonstrates that siblings do not
exist in a vacuum and that what affects their parents ultimately affects them.
For child or adolescent siblings, fear may be intensified when parents keep
information away from them in an effort to protect them from disturbing
news. If parents are taught how to communicate information in an age-appropriate way, they can provide explanations that alleviate their children's
anxiety and feelings of being left out of the family. Chapter 4 is devoted to
how to impart such information. It offers a great tip (saying, "I don't know,
but I'll find out") that helps parents buy time to figure out how to communicate in language the child can understand. Boxes with Tips for Families
emphasize central themes essential for successful intervention with siblings
and their families.

While Ms. Rector has provided thoughtful interventions, she has also
shown cultural sensitivity with ways to interact with families from different
backgrounds. In some situations, options are presented within a context

that no pressure is placed on a family to do other than their own culture permits. Ms. Rector suggests that information be given in the family's first language. Honor and respect for individuality is a theme throughout the book and most likely has led to Ms. Rector's real success with families of many cultures in a tertiary NICU setting.

A variety of professionals work in the NICU, and Ms. Rector provides some tips on roles they can take with families during the NICU experience. Other disciplines that will find this reference useful will be social service staff, child life specialists, occupational therapists, developmental specialists, and, of course, nursing staff that are in the unit during sibling visitation.

Ms. Rector gives the professional a variety of activities to help siblings participate in meaningful ways while the baby is in the NICU. Whether it is creating bedside artwork, picking balloons or photos, or making a name sign, these opportunities are inclusive activities that launch the new relationship between baby and sibling. Practical advice on learning hospital policies so as not to disappoint is included and can help families avoid hurt and aggravation.

Ms. Rector not only discusses sibling visitation but also what happens when parents leave their children to go and visit the baby in the NICU (Chapter 5). These visits may create a hardship for both parents and children for differing reasons. Transportation/parking costs, child care availability and costs, and sibling distress are some of the challenges staff in the NICU forget as they welcome a parent who comes to visit. Identifying issues with visitation and helping parents resolve them can help parents be with their baby instead of worrying about the problems surrounding NICU visits.

In Chapter 6, Ms. Rector presents early studies that show positive benefits for siblings who visit their brother or sister in the NICU. One study demonstrated a successful approach to sibling visitation, but overall research is lacking in this area. By piecing together available evidence and personal knowledge based on years of experience, Ms. Rector has written an excellent chapter on a variety of strategies to make the NICU visitation a successful experience. Further research to determine what interventions work best with a variety of age groups is definitely needed.

Chapter 7 is full of sensible activities to help children or adolescents cope with the birth of a high-risk newborn and the resulting hospitalization. In Chapter 8, Ms. Rector provides national and international sibling support groups and methods of choosing an appropriate referral based on family needs. In Chapter 9, she explores working with siblings whose mother is having multiple babies and the issues that situation will generate for the siblings and family. Chapters 10 and 11 deal with discharge and going home at length, and rightly so, because that time is fraught with tension, home preparation, learning about care, and safety.

Although it is difficult to look at the challenging aspects of life, the death of an infant must be faced in order to move forward. Babies are not forgotten, but when feelings are suppressed and ignored and siblings are not allowed to mourn, the family is suspended and unable to continue with a normal life progression. In Chapter 12, Ms. Rector looks at death straight on and shows how different age groups perceive death or express grief. She shows how rituals, ceremonies, and just saying good-bye can encourage healing.

Not to be forgotten are siblings of children who have survived the NICU to have special needs. The chronic nature of their brother's or sister's condition may mean that life at home will never be the same again and that a variety of adjustments will need to be made. The type of adaptations needed for these children is discussed in Chapter 13, and the following chapter on growing up with a sibling with special needs completes this well-rounded volume on siblings of high-risk infants.

In addition to the text, the back of the book includes resources such as suggestions and activities, Internet resources and web sites by disease or organization, sibling Internet sites, and books for siblings. This extensive resource list is compiled for further study if the reader desires more information.

Thanks to Ms. Rector's efforts, there is now a practical reference to help professionals provide support for siblings and their families before, during, and after the high-risk infant's NICU stay. Her thorough review of the literature reveals gaps in the current evidence base and may launch interest in future research. In addition, this volume is a rare combination of theory and practical application that will not be left on the bookshelf to gather dust.

Carol Turnage Carrier, M.S.N., RN, CNS
Newborn Clinical Nurse Specialist
Newborn Center, Texas Children's Hospital
Houston, Texas

Preface

The addition of a new baby is a very exciting experience for many families, but it can become frightening and confusing when the new baby develops problems and is hospitalized in the neonatal intensive care unit (NICU). Many families are interested in promoting a positive beginning to the relationship between their older children and the new baby while the baby is hospitalized in the NICU as well as following discharge. They can have numerous questions and concerns about what to tell siblings and other young relatives about the baby as well as how to support them during this experience. Some parents are unaware of the importance of sibling issues or have difficulty focusing on them, so the health care team may not be aware that some siblings are having difficulty until the situation has reached a crisis level.

Many NICUs in the United States have adopted family-centered care guidelines and have integrated families into their units. In the beginning, *family* was often defined as only the baby's parents. This has begun to change, and most units now include grandparents in their definition of family, and many also include siblings as well. In some maternity units, NICUs, and hospices, though, siblings can still be limited in their ability to participate, even when the hospitalization continues for an extended period of time. Their visits can be limited to specific times or days of the week, which may not always fit well into the family's schedule or routine. Because different families can define *family* in different ways, it can be helpful to allow parents to identify the baby's "siblings" rather than relying on an institution's definition. There may be other children such as cousins, young aunts and uncles, and friends who live in the same home as the baby or nearby and have the role of "sibling" but are not the baby's biological or adopted siblings. These children can be greatly affected by the baby's NICU hospitalization, diagnosis, or death and may need assistance and support to cope with these experiences.

The members of the health care team who are primarily responsible for assisting families with sibling issues can vary during different aspects of this experience. Child life specialists and some social workers have training and experience in this area, but these professionals may not always be available. All members of the health care team who have contact with siblings during different aspects of this experience can benefit from having some knowledge of sibling issues. What they say and do and how they interact with siblings has the potential to affect how siblings may respond to the baby's hospitalization. Siblings can also be influenced by the perceptions and coping styles of other family members. This can be affected by issues such as the family's cultural and religious background, their previous experiences with the health care system, their available support systems, parental educational background, and their financial resources.

This book was written to help increase the amount of sibling information available for professionals who work with high-risk infants and their families. Not every suggestion will be applicable for every sibling or family or for every institution. Interventions that work well for one sibling and family may not work well for others. Also, the interventions that work best for a sibling or family can change over time, especially as the sibling grows and moves through different developmental stages and as the baby's condition changes. The information and research on some of these issues tend to be spotty and dated. Even though this has changed in some areas, there continues to be a great need for updated information and research in several areas. Siblings are important family members, and more information is needed on how to assist and support them throughout the different aspects of this experience.

Due to the importance of continuity and coordination of care, including not only professionals who interact with siblings and their families while the baby is in the NICU but also those who will interact with families prior to the baby's birth and after the baby has been discharged is important. Examples of professionals who could benefit from this information include various members of the health care team in the high-risk maternity unit and NICU, home care staff, high-risk obstetricians, family pediatricians, and individuals at the siblings' schools, as well as other individuals who assist and support these siblings and their families.

*To the babies hospitalized in the NICU
and their big brothers and sisters;
to my family, who has helped
me to accomplish my goals and dreams; and
to Carol Turnage Carrier for her assistance,
encouragement, and support*

I

The Developmental Perspective

Siblings Across the Age Span

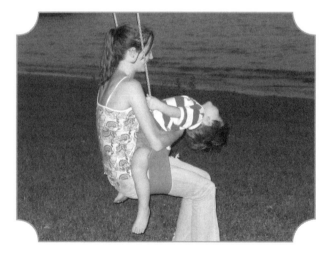

The way children respond to their mother's pregnancy and the birth of a new brother or sister depends on their developmental level, maturity, temperament, past experiences, support systems, family dynamics, and cultural and religious beliefs. Children at the same developmental level tend to have some of the same characteristics that can help them understand and cope with the birth of a new sibling. This chapter is organized by developmental level to highlight the characteristics of siblings at certain ages. Although families may know how their children have coped with stressful situations in the past, they can often benefit from information specific to this particular experience.

OLDER INFANT SIBLINGS

Some babies in the NICU have siblings who are older infants (around 6–12 months of age). Their families have experienced two pregnancies and births in a short period, which can increase their stress and reduce their coping and financial resources. Some of these families are still recovering from their previous pregnancy and birth experiences, especially if these events were difficult or high risk, which can affect how they may cope with their current situation. For many older infant siblings, their mother's pregnancy occurred shortly after they were born, which may have influenced how their mother was able to interact or care for them, especially if the new pregnancy was high risk.

Older infant siblings depend heavily on their families and tend to have had limited experiences without them. They are often sensitive to changes in their routine as well as to changes in their parents' stress level and emotional reactions, which often occur during this time. Families may see increased crying, clinginess, and difficulty separating from parents. These siblings benefit most from consistent caregivers who are familiar with them and their routines and who are able to understand their vocalizations and gestures. It is also important that these caregivers are aware of safety issues. Older infants are beginning to explore their environment and are learning to crawl, cruise around furniture, and possibly take their first independent steps. All of their environments should be safe and childproof.

If they are separated from their parents for an extended time, some older infant siblings may begin to form strong attachments to their consistent caregiver and turn to that individual for comfort and to get their needs met, even in their parents' presence. This can be upsetting for many parents and, for some, devastating. Some parents may even feel that they have failed as parents. They need to be assured that their child's behavior does not necessarily reflect a failure but can actually be viewed as a success! They have chosen a caregiver who is able to provide the loving care their child needs in their absence. After family life begins to settle down and parents are able to spend more time with their child on a consistent basis, the sibling will once again begin to look to them for his or her physical, emotional, and support needs. Even though they have provided excellent caregivers, parents still need to spend quality time with older infant siblings as often as possible.

TODDLER SIBLINGS

Toddler siblings (around 1–3 years of age) can recognize additional stress and changes in daily routines that often occur in families during this time. Fiese (2002) reported that familiar routines can help reduce stress during times of uncertainty. Continuing these routines can help provide toddlers with the comfort, stability, and security they need to help them cope with aspects of their family's new situation. Consistent caregivers can also provide comfort, stability, and security, but it is important to consider this issue from the toddler's perspective. Caregivers should be individuals with whom the toddler is familiar, rather than individuals who are familiar with the toddler but whom the toddler does not remember.

The Rosado family asked a grandmother who had last seen their 18-month-old daughter, Rose, at Christmas 6 months earlier, to stay with her while they spent time with the baby in the NICU. Rose did not remember her grandmother from their previous meeting, and due to the stress surrounding the baby's early arrival and NICU admission, no one had thought to help her become better acquainted. As a result, Rose had extreme difficulty reconnecting with her grandmother. When her mother left to visit the baby, Rose actively cried for long periods. When it became evident that her parents were not going to return, she stopped crying and began to withdraw.

Mrs. Yee had been diagnosed with a high-risk pregnancy, and her family was told that the baby would probably have to spend time in the NICU. Mr. and Mrs. Yee began to prepare their first child, Thomas (age 20 months), for his grandmother's arrival by looking through family photographs and talking about his grandmother on a regular basis. They also purchased extra copies of Thomas's favorite storybooks, mailed them to his grandmother, and asked her to videotape herself reading them for "Grandma's storytime." She not only mailed back the videotapes but also sent periodic surprises. By the time Thomas's grandmother arrived, his parents had integrated Grandma's storytime into his bedtime routine, and he had become excited about seeing his grandma. This toddler sibling was able to quickly make a positive connection with his grandmother. When his parents left to visit his baby brother, Thomas cried and showed distress but was able to be comforted and supported by his grandmother until their return.

The Porters were expecting a healthy, full-term baby and were surprised when told that their baby needed to be admitted to the NICU immediately after his birth. With the mother in one hospital, the baby in another, and the father going back and forth between them, the Porters needed to find additional care quickly for their 2-year-old daughter, Stephanie. She was currently staying with her baby sitter, who was also keeping Stephanie overnight as a favor to the Porters, but the baby sitter was unable to care for Stephanie on a long-term basis. An aunt was available to fly in and care for Stephanie but had not seen her in several months. Mrs. Porter jotted down a list of important information, such as Stephanie's daily routine, favorite foods, toys and books, and security items. She also arranged for the aunt to spend time with the baby sitter and Stephanie together. This arrangement gave Stephanie the opportunity to become reacquainted with her aunt in the presence of someone with whom she was familiar. It also allowed time for the aunt and baby sitter to become acquainted and to share information and support regarding Stephanie.

Tip for Families

It is important to share information about siblings' routines with their familiar, consistent caregivers so that caregivers can help the siblings cope with the family's situation.

Coping

Toddler siblings often utilize regression to cope with a variety of stressful situations. Volling (2005) reported that siblings sometimes demonstrate a developmental setback when a new baby is added to their family. Families may need reassurance that the setback is usually temporary. The duration often depends on the child and the different issues he or she may be coping with at the time.

Toddlers tend to have limited language skills and may use their behaviors as a way to cope and to express themselves. It is often beneficial to try to determine the reason for these behaviors. This can be difficult and frustrating for families, especially while they are coping with the mother's or baby's issues or both. Many families need assistance translating their children's behaviors.

The Gonzalez family had a premature baby admitted to the hospital and a 22-month-old daughter, Marisol, at home. Mr. and Mrs. Gonzalez attempted to maintain Marisol's daily routine by continuing with her regular baby sitter while Mrs. Gonzalez spent time with the baby during the day. They also tried to continue their routine of a family meal together and Marisol's bedtime routine before returning to the hospital to see the baby in the evening. Mr. and Mrs. Gonzalez began to receive reports from the baby sitter that Marisol was having increased periods of distress during the day as well as difficulty interacting with the other children the baby sitter was caring for. Marisol started to refuse to eat during the family meal, making the once-enjoyable family routine begin to resemble a battle. At bedtime, she began to cry more and get out of bed more often. She believed that her parents loved the new baby more than they loved her, but she did not have the verbal skills to express her feelings.

Hector, who was a 30-month-old sibling, was having increased temper tantrums at home, and his parents had received reports of negative behavior from his mother's day out teacher. One afternoon while playing with his trucks with his father, Hector stated that the smallest truck was bad and had to stay in another garage. When his father asked him why he thought the smallest truck was bad, his response was because the smallest truck had to go the hospital. Hector wanted to spend more time with his mamá and papa and thought being "bad" might be a way to accomplish this because it had worked for his baby sister. Hector thought his baby sister was in the NICU because she had done something bad. Several days ago, he had overheard his papa tell his abuela something about the baby, "bad," and the hospital.

Tip for Families

It is best to wait until the family's stress level is reduced and consistent routines have returned before introducing new developmental tasks to toddler siblings. Examples might be moving to a "big kid" bed, weaning from the bottle or breast, potty training, or starting center-based child care or mother's day out. These developmental issues can be difficult for toddlers under the best of circumstances but can be even more difficult when the family is stressed.

Participation in the Baby's Care

Providing opportunities for toddler siblings to participate in the baby's care in the hospital and home environments can help them learn how to interact safely with the baby and begin to accept the baby as a member of the family. Some toddler siblings may want to be involved with the baby, whereas others may ignore all aspects of the baby. Even though toddler siblings are young, there are still ways to involve them in the baby's care. For instance, they could hand the caregiver items for the baby, such as diapers; help pick out the baby's clothes, hats, or socks; or choose toys and other items they think the baby might enjoy. Toddlers can also benefit from helping to care for their mother on bed rest by taking her snacks, helping to decorate her bed space for holidays, and playing games with her.

PRESCHOOL SIBLINGS

Preschool siblings (around 3–5 years of age) tend to view the hospitalization of the baby in various ways. They may believe they have caused some aspects of the situation because of something they said, did, thought, wished, or prayed for. There is also the potential for preschool siblings to believe they have caused the additional stress or sadness in their family; their mother's high-risk pregnancy or bed rest; or the baby's hospitalization, diagnosis, or death.

Three-year-old Tara was aware that her parents were worried since her baby brother's birth and admission to the hospital. She had even seen them cry a few times when they didn't know she was looking. She believed that she had caused her parents to cry because of her "bad" behavior at her grandmother's house the night her baby brother was born. Tara had heard her grandmother and father talking about it when he came to pick her up.

Olivia, a 4-year-old big sister, was tired of her mother being on bed rest and told her prekindergarten teacher that she was not going to have a new baby at her house. When her baby sister was admitted to the NICU instead of coming home, Olivia believed it was her fault.

Preschool siblings may also believe that the next time they are sick, they will need to go to the hospital just as the baby or possibly their mother had.

Carlos, a 3-year-old sibling, got a stomachache after raiding his grandmother's cookie jar. He began to worry that he would have to go to the hospital like the baby had. He was especially afraid that his parents would leave him there alone overnight, just as they did with the baby. Carlos was also afraid of the dark and worried that he would not be able to take his flashlight. The more he worried, the more upset his stomach became, until he finally vomited and his

family learned about the cookies. They became angry, yelled at him, and sent him to his room to think about what he had done. All he could think about was that he was going to the hospital like the baby and that he would be alone.

Four-year-old William slid out of a tree and scraped his knee and elbow on the way down. He was afraid to tell his father because he thought he would have to go to the doctor and then to the hospital like his mother had. A few weeks ago, his mother had left him with his baby sitter while she went to the doctor and was going to pick him up after his favorite cartoon, but she did not come home until the baby was born. William's father learned about the scrapes that night while giving him a bath and asked him why he had not mentioned them earlier. William's father assured him that his scrapes could be treated at home. He also informed him that most children do not need to go to the hospital, but that if he ever did, his mommy or daddy would always be there.

Rozdilsky (2005) discussed that preschoolers have the potential to view hospitalization as punishment. This view is more likely to occur if they have been told that if they misbehave, they will be given a shot, will have to stay in the hospital, or that their parents will tell the doctor.

Jacinta's parents told her she could not have a soft drink out of the machine near the NICU waiting room. When she began to realize that her parents really meant no, the 3-year-old started to cry. Her stressed parents warned her that if she did not stop crying, they would tell the doctor and she would have to stay in the hospital with the babies. Later that night as she was putting her baby dolls to bed, Jacinta told them that if they were bad, they would have to go to the hospital and stay with her baby sister.

Xavier (age 4 years) could not sit still and began running up and down the hallways outside the NICU. His mother loudly informed him that if he did not stop, she would tell the doctor to give him a big shot. A few minutes later, the baby's physician walked up to the family to give them an update on their baby's progress. Xavier took one look at him and began to scream "No shots!" and then turned and ran in the other direction.

Providing accurate and developmentally appropriate explanations frequently, as well as opportunities to visit the mother and baby in the hospital, can help reduce misunderstandings and misconceptions among preschool siblings. Many have had little or no experience with the hospital environment and may have difficulty visualizing where their mother and the baby are.

Routines and Caregivers

Familiar, consistent routines and familiar, consistent caregivers can help support preschool siblings. Changes in their routines signal that something different or unusual has happened in their family. Familiar routines help them understand and recognize the rhythm of their day. When their routines change, it can be difficult for them to cope. The amount of change children are able to tolerate varies. Families that have difficulty maintaining siblings' routines during this time may need support. Sharing information such as preschool siblings' routines, likes and dislikes, and coping strategies with familiar, consistent caregivers can help caregivers ease siblings' fears and frustrations.

Preschool siblings often use parents and other important adults as role models for coping during stressful experiences. They may look to these individuals for support and for appropriate ways to respond in unfamiliar situations. Even when preschoolers appear not to be paying attention to what is going on around them, they are often closely observing the behavior of these adults. They may also begin to view the adults they encounter in preschool, mother's day out, playgroups, center-based child care, or organized sports as role models.

Tip for Families

It can be helpful to talk about the family's situation with siblings' other caregivers, such as teachers and coaches, and ask them to share any behavior changes or coping issues they might observe.

When possible, parents should spend special time with preschool siblings so that they will feel included in their family's experience and understand that they have not been replaced by the baby. Spending special time may be more difficult in some families than in others, especially in those that have more than one older sibling. Some families have managed to make special time a part of their regular family routines, such as grocery shopping, washing the car, folding laundry, or cooking a simple recipe together.

Coping

Like toddlers, many preschool siblings utilize regression to cope with stressful experiences. Volling (2005) reported that siblings may demonstrate developmental setbacks in response to a new sibling. These setbacks are often temporary, although the length of time can depend on issues related to the individual sibling and situation. Preschool siblings tend to respond better when their "big girl" or "big boy" behaviors are positively reinforced rather than when their regressive behaviors are punished or ridiculed. Sawicki (1997) noted that some of these behaviors may be the older sibling's attempt to imitate the baby's behaviors. Giving preschool siblings opportunities to experiment with the baby's belongings as well as a chance to try out the baby's role may, over time, allow them to recognize the advantages of being a "big boy" or "big girl."

Another way preschool siblings may cope is through attention-seeking behaviors. These behaviors usually occur when the family's attention is directed elsewhere, such as after the baby's birth or discharge from the hospital. These "watch me" or "look at me" behaviors are unintentional ways to draw attention away from the baby and toward themselves. Families should be cautioned about what behaviors they are reinforcing during this time. Overwhelmed parents may misunderstand why their child is misbehaving and consistently punish him or her for it, which provides the sibling with the parents' attention, even though the attention may be negative. The behavior often escalates, which can frustrate parents even further and lead to even more punishment. In these situations, parents should be encouraged to pay attention to the sibling's positive behaviors and ignore as many of the negative behaviors as possible.

Fantasy Play

Fantasy play can help preschoolers better understand and successfully cope with new experiences. Kramer (1996) stated that preschool siblings who used fantasy play to cope with the birth of healthy, full-term babies were reported by their mothers as having a more positive relationship with the baby. As the new experience changes, the amount and type of fantasy play that siblings participate in may also change. Kramer and Schafer-Hernan (1994) reported that the amount of fantasy play that siblings engaged in was related to the amount of stress they felt during specific aspects of the experience. They also noted that fantasy play with a friend decreased around the time the baby was born and then returned to prebirth levels when the baby was about 3 months old. Special materials to facilitate fantasy play can be beneficial for preschool siblings but are not always necessary for fantasy play to take place.

Three-year-old Jessie was helping her mother set the table and began to play with the silverware. She divided the silverware into family groups. She identified the knives as the daddies, because they were the tallest; the forks as the mommies, because they were the second tallest; the spoons as the big sisters,

because they were used to eat ice cream, which was her favorite; and the salad forks as the babies, because they were smaller than the other forks. As her mother finished preparing dinner, Jessie sat at the table and played with her silverware families.

Sam, age 3, played with some pencils while helping his father at his desk. During his play, he sorted out the pencils to represent different members of his family. He put the mama, papa, big sister, and big brother pencils in one pencil holder and called it their house. He put the smallest pencil, which he called the baby, in a separate pencil holder and said that the pencil was in the hospital because it was sick. He continued to play with his pencil family until his father completed his work and was ready to play catch outside.

Tip for Families

When adults engage in fantasy play with children, it is important to allow the child to be in charge of the play and for the adult to follow the child's lead.

Participation in the Baby's Care

Many preschool siblings enjoy participating in different aspects of expecting and having a new baby, such as helping care for their mother on bed rest or being involved in the baby's care. Their attempts to help should be recognized and appreciated or, if they are not appropriate, gently redirected. Providing multiple opportunities for involvement can help make siblings feel that they are important members of their family. Ways to involve these siblings in the baby's care in the hospital and home environments include handing adult caregivers items such as diapers and blankets; picking out the baby's clothes for the day; and interacting with the baby, such as touching and kissing, as well as talking, singing, and playing with the baby. Preschool siblings can also be involved in the baby's medical care, for example, by entertaining or distracting the baby while the adult provides medical care.

SCHOOL-AGE SIBLINGS

Like preschoolers, school-age siblings (around 5–10 years of age) may believe that they have caused their mother's or the baby's difficulties and possibly some of the changes in their home environment. They, too, can benefit from age-appropriate explanations, which can help clarify any misunderstandings or misconceptions they might have. Because school-age children tend to be concrete thinkers, they can utilize simple diagrams or anatomy books to help them better understand their mother's and the baby's diagnoses and issues.

Routines and Caregivers

As with toddler and preschool siblings, maintaining familiar, consistent caregivers and familiar family routines can help provide school-age siblings with support and stability. The amount of consistency siblings require varies. In difficult situations, families may need assistance in finding ways to provide consistency for siblings.

Seven-year-old Alina was excited about becoming a big sister in the spring and enjoyed helping her parents get ready for the baby at home. Along the way, however, her mother had to be hospitalized with pregnancy complications. Her father was spending less time at home because he was visiting his wife in the hospital and working overtime to help pay the unexpected medical bills.

Alina's parents talked with several of her friends' parents and arranged for a different family to care for her each day of the week in order not to burden any one family. They began to receive reports from Alina's teacher that she was having difficulty with some of her work and was not interacting with the other children as she had in the past. The families reported that Alina seemed withdrawn and was not eating.

Alina's mother met with the family's social worker, who recommended choosing one family, preferably the one with which Alina was most comfortable, and providing them with information on daily routines as well as likes and dislikes. She also discussed the possibility of Dad stopping by for dinner and participating in Alina's bedtime routine on his way from work to the hospital to visit Mom. The social worker also suggested that Alina's parents offer to support the other family in the future during their own possible crisis or to watch their children whenever the parents wished to spend time alone.

Ms. Amanda discussed with the neonatal child life specialist that her 8-year-old daughter, Ruby, was having a hard time dealing with the baby's admission to the NICU. They discussed the changes that Ruby had experienced since the baby's admission as well as during her mother's pregnancy. Ms. Amanda reported that she had relaxed a number of the rules at home as well as the family's routines. She thought that Ruby needed a break and that this was the best way to do it. The neonatal child life specialist shared the importance of maintaining familiar routines, especially during times of stress.

Kadeem, age 8, liked the idea of becoming a big brother but repeatedly stated that he would never change the baby's diapers. He stayed at his best friend's house while his parents went to the hospital to have the baby. Unfortunately, the baby had a problem and had to be admitted to a hospital several hundred miles away. Kadeem's mother was still recovering from the birth, and his father needed to be with the baby, so they quickly arranged for Kadeem to continue to stay with his best friend's family.

Before leaving, Kadeem's father gave the friend's family a house key so that his son could get clothes and other items as needed. He also exchanged telephone numbers and e-mail addresses with the family to maintain contact while he was away. The best friend's mother and Kadeem's teacher reported some changes in his behavior but that he responded well to support and was able to continue with his regular activities.

Support

School-age siblings participate in many events and activities outside of their family. Although their parents continue to be their primary source of support during the experience of a new baby, some school-age siblings may utilize other individuals as well, such as teachers, coaches, scout leaders, baby sitters, or neighbors. Wallinga and Skeen (1996) reported that teachers can become important, consistent individuals in children's lives when a sibling is hospitalized. When teachers are informed of the baby's hospitalization, they can help support siblings and communicate possible problems to parents. Wallinga and Skeen also reported that teachers can help reinforce children's understanding of the new situation and can help them share information with their peers.

Some parents may be tempted to communicate information to teachers without consulting the child. Although some siblings may not have a problem with this, others will want a say in what information will be shared with their teachers, as well as with their friends and classmates. Allowing input from siblings has the added benefit of making siblings feel included.

Coping

Some school-age siblings may regress, but as with younger siblings, regression will diminish with time. Rather than punishing or ridiculing siblings for their regressive behaviors, families and members of the health care team should try to reinforce their age-appropriate behaviors.

Six-year-old Dory began to wet the bed after the birth and admission of her baby sister to the NICU. This was more than her stressed parents could handle.

They began to call her a baby and told her she needed to grow up. Several days later, Dory's teacher reported that she was having similar accidents at school.

Nina, age 6, started to wet the bed after her baby brother was admitted to the NICU. Her parents assured her that this sometimes happens to big sisters and that it was "no big deal." They provided several aids, such as a plastic sheet on her bed, special underpants for nighttime, and a sleeping bag on the floor in her room so that she would always have a dry place to sleep. They further assured her that these items were available whenever she needed them, even in the middle of the night. Nina continued to wet the bed periodically for several weeks and then stopped entirely.

Some school-age siblings may cope with the family's new situation by trying to be the perfect child. These siblings can easily be overlooked because they are not causing problems or because adults believe they are coping well and do not need additional support. Some siblings may believe they need to be perfect due to feelings of guilt that they have caused some of the stress in their family. They may also become overly upset when they make mistakes or when things do not go exactly right.

Participation in the Baby's Care

Like many school-age siblings of healthy, full-term babies who want to be involved in their family's pregnancy and in the baby's care, school-age siblings of babies admitted to the NICU may also wish to be involved. Their level of involvement will depend on the baby's and mother's medical conditions and parents' comfort levels. Families may need assistance and support on ways to successfully adapt caregiving issues and routines so that school-age siblings can be involved in different aspects of their mother's and the baby's care in the NICU and home environments. School-age siblings may enjoy helping their family purchase special items for the baby as well as holding and interacting with their new brother or sister. Also, depending on the baby's nutritional needs, they may be able to help with feedings. They can also become experts at providing distraction during certain medical treatments that may be difficult for the baby. Sibling participation in the baby's care should be reviewed periodically on the basis of changes in the mother's and baby's condition and changes in the sibling's abilities and interest.

PRETEEN SIBLINGS

Preteen siblings (around 10–13 years of age) are able to understand the perspective of others better than younger siblings can. They may attempt to conceal their concerns and emotions in an effort to protect their parents. They may even be told by well-meaning family members and friends that they need to be strong for their parents.

Some begin to accept or assume additional responsibilities or household tasks that they may or may not be ready to take on, sometimes due to inadequate family resources or support and the need for additional assistance during this time. Some families expect siblings to accept these added responsibilities, whereas preteens in other families gradually take on additional tasks without their parents being aware that it has occurred. If these responsibilities continue for an extended period, however, preteen siblings may have less time for activities that promote their own growth and development. On the other hand, performing additional responsibilities provides preteens with positive benefits, such as contributing to their family as a team player and becoming more self-sufficient.

Some families need to be reminded that preteen siblings already have an important job—that of growing into a competent adult—and that they should continue to have opportunities to do so. Parents may also need help in locating assistance they have not yet considered. One example might be utilizing a teenager in the neighborhood who is willing to work for a small fee or who needs community service hours for graduation. This individual might be able to assist with a variety of chores, such as yard work, house cleaning, cooking, laundry, or pet care.

Routines and Caregivers

Familiar, consistent caregivers and routines as well as familiar environments continue to be important issues for many preteens. Those who are entering puberty will need the support of familiar caregivers while their parents are away. Privacy is also typically important to preteens, and it can be difficult for them if they are staying somewhere other than their own home. Preteens often spend more time with their friends, as peer relationships become increasingly important during these years. If they are staying somewhere away from their peer group, they may experience difficulty. Families may need to be reminded about the importance of being able to maintain contact with friends.

Support

Many preteens are making the move to middle school or junior high, and this transition can be difficult for them. Parents who are coping with a high-risk pregnancy or a baby in the NICU will have less time and energy to assist them with this transition. Because they may be worrying about issues at home or the hospital, preteens may have difficultly not only concentrating in school, but also completing homework assignments and studying for tests in a timely fashion. It may be helpful for families and siblings to share information with important individuals at school, such as the counselor, homeroom teacher, or other teachers. These individuals may be able to help support siblings and share information with parents when needed.

> **Tip for Families**
>
> Preteen siblings may want to have a primary role in what is communicated to individuals at their school. If their input is ignored, they can feel angry and upset.

Participation in the Baby's Care

Some preteen siblings may want to participate in their mother's and the baby's care. They can often benefit from opportunities to be involved in both the hospital and home environments. Issues such as the sibling's interest level, the mother's and the baby's medical conditions, and parents' comfort levels should be considered. Preteens will also often benefit from information on infant safety and developmental issues.

ADOLESCENT SIBLINGS

Adolescent siblings (around 13–18 years of age) can misunderstand aspects of their mother's or the baby's condition but may hesitate to ask for clarification because they do not want to appear unintelligent in front of others. They may discuss some of their concerns with their friends, who may or may not provide accurate information or advice. Some adolescents benefit from printed information or information found on web sites, although it is important to check with parents before any information is shared with them. If web site addresses are provided, adolescents may also need tips on Internet safety as well as how to critically review health information found on the Internet (see Resources at the end of the book).

Support

As with preteen siblings, adolescent siblings can be asked to assume additional household responsibilities. These responsibilities can be time consuming and can affect the available time adolescent siblings have to participate in school and peer activities. These activities assist siblings with their coping abilities and can also promote their growth and development. Some families may need assistance in considering new resources, such as their church, their children's schools, neighbors, or even a student from a local university. Adolescents, however, can gain positive benefits from these additional responsibilities, such as contributing to their family, learning new skills, and becoming more self-sufficient.

Adolescents are usually in high school and may be involved in a variety of extracurricular activities. During difficult times, however, siblings' home

Tip for Families

Families may want to consider including adolescent siblings in both formal and informal family meetings with the health care team. This involvement can help them gain a better understanding of the baby's issues and feel as if they are important team members. Follow-up should be provided to reinforce information and to assist with misunderstandings and misconceptions.

routines can change, making it harder for them to study for tests and complete homework assignments. There may even be times when they have to miss school. Also, parents may be less available for assistance and support. Sharing information with teachers and counselors can help them support siblings and assist them with schoolwork and other issues.

Participation in the Baby's Care

Adolescent siblings can benefit from opportunities to be involved in the baby's care in the NICU and home environments. Those who participate in school and extracurricular activities or have part-time jobs may need to schedule their involvement around these events. Many adolescent siblings are able to be involved in aspects of the baby's medical care, but as with other age groups, it will depend on the complexity of care as well as parents' comfort levels.

ADULT SIBLINGS

A few babies in the NICU have adult siblings (18 years of age or older). Adult siblings tend to have more resources for information and support than younger siblings. They can often utilize resources that were written for parents, and their social circles typically increase as they move to university and job environments. Whether these siblings live in the same town as their parents or across the country, they still have a need for information. Adult siblings can often benefit from suggestions for web sites and other resources (see Resources at the end of the book). They may also desire opportunities to participate in formal meetings with the health care team. Siblings who live far away may benefit from visits scheduled in advance so that they have adequate time to make travel arrangements. If travel is not an option, they might consider communicating with members of the health care team by telephone or by e-mail after permission has been received from the parents.

Adult siblings who wish to participate in aspects of the NICU experience should be provided with opportunities to spend time in the hospital and home environments. Their involvement may be affected by such issues as where they live, their occupation, and, if applicable, their own family life.

CONCLUSION

Siblings' developmental level will affect how siblings respond to their mother's pregnancy and the baby's hospitalization. It can also influence the information and support siblings will need to help them cope. Although siblings at the same developmental level can have many of the same characteristics, each sibling is an individual and will cope with this experience in his or her own way. Families may need extra assistance when two or more siblings have very different coping styles or when a sibling's coping changes as he or she continues to grow and develop.

The High-Risk Pregnancy

The Big Brother's and Sister's Perspective

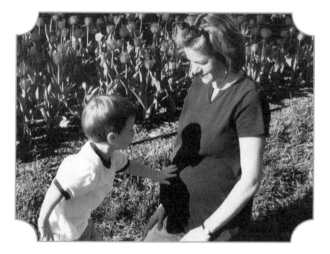

Prenatal examinations, tests, and assessments can provide families with helpful information, such as the baby's sex or the need to plan for multiples. Obstetricians and other physicians may recommend assessments or tests for possible health problems for the mother or to check for problems or abnormalities in the fetus. The anticipation or expectation of a problem is often frightening and overwhelming for families. If a problem is suspected or diagnosed, the family's initial birth plan may no longer be applicable, and they may need assistance from their health care team to develop a new one. They also may need help coping with the differences between this pregnancy and birth experience and previous pregnancies and birth experiences in their family.

DISCUSSING THE HIGH-RISK PREGNANCY WITH SIBLINGS

Parents may not understand or accept all of the information they have been given, which can make it difficult for them to share it with other family members. They may be unsure of what to tell their children when a complication is diagnosed or suspected during the pregnancy and may require assistance and support when they share information with them. Some parents may decide not to talk with their children in an attempt to protect them. They may believe that sharing information will overwhelm or frighten them. Parents may receive different information from different physicians, making it difficult for them to know what to tell their children. They may decide to wait until after the baby is born and they are more certain about the baby's diagnosis and outcome before they talk with their children about the baby's issues. Some parents may decide not to share information with their children for cultural reasons. They should be supported even if their decision differs from the health care team's.

Ms. Jenkins, her mother, and her 5-year-old daughter, Brianna, were anticipating the addition of a new baby to their family. During a routine visit with her doctor, Ms. Jenkins learned that the baby had a major heart defect and would need surgery soon after birth. She began to be followed more closely by the doctor and was provided with information about the surgical procedure. Ms. Jenkins and her mother had a great deal of difficulty understanding this information and tended to rely on what the physicians recommended. When the health care team asked about sharing information with Brianna, Ms. Jenkins and her mother were adamant that they did not want her to know about the baby's heart defect. When questioned further, they reported that they felt it was too much for Brianna to understand. Also, they did not want her to worry about the baby and disrupt her year in kindergarten.

The Chin family was anticipating the birth of twins. During a scheduled pre-natal ultrasound, they learned that one of the twins had a significant myelomeningocele. They were referred to several specialists who provided them with different options for treatment. This added to their confusion about the best course of treatment for their baby. They also had difficulty sifting through all of the information to figure out what to tell their 3-year-old daughter, Lien, and 8-year-old daughter, An. Because of this, they decided to wait until the twins were born before they discussed the myelomeningocele with their daughters. Mr. and Mrs. Chin were unaware their daughters were receiving information in other ways, such as from conversations going on around them, changes in their routine, and changes in the family stress level.

The Navarro family was visiting the United States from Panama and planned to return to Panama when Mr. Navarro completed specialized training for his job. They were expecting their fourth child, who was diagnosed with a gastroschisis, or an opening in the abdominal wall. Mr. and Mrs. Navarro did not want to discuss the possibility of preparing their 6-year-old twins, Manuel and Miguel, and 8-year-old daughter Mercedes for the baby's NICU admission and need for surgery. Mrs. Navarro explained, "That's not how we do it where we are from." The social worker and child life specialist let Mr. and Mrs. Navarro know that they were available to provide assistance and support on this issue if they needed it in the future. They also provided information on additional ways to support the Navarro children in Spanish, the family's primary language.

Tip for Families

Many siblings are able to recognize when their family is facing a difficult situation because of changes in their family's routines and stress levels. If information is not shared with them in a developmentally appropriate manner, siblings may believe that they have somehow caused the recent changes they are observing in their family.

Many children begin to form a relationship with the baby during their mother's pregnancy as they discuss the new baby with family members, watch their mother's belly grow, talk to the baby as they snuggle beside their mother, feel the baby kick, or help choose the baby's name. Siblings' developmental level should be considered when including them in aspects of the pregnancy and when sharing information with them. Even young siblings can often understand that the baby will need extra help after it is born.

Younger Siblings

Preschool and school-age siblings are often ready for anatomical information, such as which body part or body system is affected. They can benefit from being included in a few of their mother's prenatal visits, where they can listen to the baby's heartbeat, help to measure their mother's belly, or look at the baby's ultrasounds. Looking at their own baby pictures or videos and discussing some of their experiences as a baby with other family members may also be beneficial for young siblings. It can help prepare them for the baby's small size and the amount of care the baby will need from their parents.

Older Siblings

Preteen and adolescent siblings tend to benefit from more detailed explanations, but it is important to recognize that they can have misconceptions about human anatomy and physiology, especially around pregnancy and reproductive issues. They might be receiving information about sexual and pregnancy issues from their friends, which may not always be accurate. In addition, scheduling conflicts with school and other activities may prevent some preteens and adolescents from participating in their mother's prenatal visits. Visits can also be uncomfortable or embarrassing for some older siblings, particularly for preteen and adolescent boys, if they believe that private body parts or sexual issues will be discussed.

MATERNAL BED REST

Maternal bed rest during pregnancy can be a difficult experience for many families. Maloni, Brezinski-Tomasi, and Johnson (2001) discussed that having a mother on bed rest can affect every member of the family. They also reported that young siblings often had difficulty understanding why their mother was unable to care for them as she did in the past, or if their mother was hospitalized, why she was away from home. Explanations should take into account siblings' developmental level as well as their past experiences.

Toddlers are egocentric, making it difficult for them to put the needs of others before their own. To them, bed rest may seem like a nap, where one rests for a while and then gets up and continues with the day. Therefore, toddlers may not understand why their mother is unable to get up and care for them as she has in the past.

Preschool siblings are better able to understand that their mother needs to stay in bed to rest and to help the unborn baby grow, but they can experience difficulty as bed rest continues for an extended period. Preschoolers also tend to have a limited understanding of the concept of time, so it can be helpful to tie the anticipated end of bed rest to holidays or seasons of the year. It is a good idea to reassure preschool siblings about who will be available to help care for them while their mother is on bed rest and to tell them that they can assist this individual in caring for their mother. If their mother is on bed rest in the hospital, they should be assured that they can call and visit on a regular basis.

Separation from their mother is a stressful event for many preschool siblings. Some may blame the unborn baby for the mother being on bed rest and begin to resent the baby. If this occurs, scheduling regular times for them to play and interact with their mother can be helpful. How bed rest is described to preschool siblings is also important. Families may want to consider describing it as a way for the family to work together and help each other, or a way to spend special time with their mother rather than as a way to help the unborn baby.

School-age siblings also need to be reassured about the end of bed rest. They tend to have a better understanding of time, but it still can be helpful to tie the anticipated end of bed rest to holidays or seasons. They can also benefit from information about their mother's and the unborn baby's progress, as well as having their questions and concerns addressed. Even though they are beginning to have more experiences outside of their family, school-age siblings can have difficulty coping when their mother is hospitalized on bed rest for an extended time. They should be given opportunities to call and visit on a regular basis.

Preteens and adolescents are able to understand the reason for their mother's bed rest, and some may be very concerned about their mother and the unborn baby. Providing an atmosphere of open communication allows them to continue to ask questions and share concerns as needed. If their mother is on bed rest in the hospital, older siblings should be assured that they will be able to maintain frequent contact with their mother through telephone calls, e-mail, and visits. Because mothers on bed rest can miss siblings' extracurricular activities, important events should be taped, if possible, and the family should have a special "viewing party" at home or at the hospital with Mom following the event.

Peer relationships are very important to preteens and adolescents, but many siblings also enjoy spending time with their families, including their parents. Some siblings may enjoy spending special time with their mother while she is on bed rest. They may engage in special activities, such as scrapbooking or knitting, or old favorites, such as board games or jigsaw puzzles. Some siblings and their mothers may enjoy looking on-line for possible college choices or occupational opportunities. In some families, the preteen or adolescent sibling may take on the role of teacher and help their mother become more proficient in the use of her computer, cell phone, or MP3 player.

Familiar Routines

Maintaining family routines and rituals during the mother's bed rest can help reduce stress and improve coping for the entire family. Families may want to consider adapting some of their routines and rituals to involve the mother on bed rest. For example, if the family has dinner every night at the dining room table, this routine could be adapted so that the family eats at a card table at the mother's bedside or has a picnic on a blanket on the floor near her bed. At Christmas, if the family traditionally has one large tree in the family room, they may want to adapt this ritual into having two smaller trees—one for the family room and one near the mother's bedside. The family can then decide which ornaments will go on which tree. Perhaps the next Christmas, the new big brothers and sisters would like to have a small Christmas tree in their room to help signify that they are "big boys" or "big girls" compared with the new baby.

Tip for Families

Sharing information about family routines and rituals with siblings' caregivers can help them better assist parents in continuing these important parts of family life while the mother is on bed rest.

Familiar, Consistent Caregivers

Familiar, consistent caregivers can be comforting, reassuring, and supportive for children during times of stress. Locating these caregivers, however, can be difficult for some families. Maloni et al. (2001) reported that families are sometimes forced to utilize a patchwork of caregivers, care provided by the mother (even though she may be on bed rest), or both. Providing support and assistance to families during this time may help them find sources for child care they may not have considered. The family's child care plan should also be periodically reviewed while the mother is on bed rest to make sure it is still effective.

Mothers continue to be parents even when they are on bed rest. Maloni et al. (2001) reported that it was difficult for mothers to see their children begin to look to others for comfort and to get their needs met. Mothers can benefit by remaining involved in aspects of their children's life and interacting with them as much as possible. Opportunities might include playing and reading stories with younger siblings and letting them help decorate the bed rest environment for different holidays and seasons. Older siblings might enjoy sharing time watching DVDs, playing video and computer games, and shopping on-line.

Some individuals may attempt to protect the mother on bed rest by taking over part of her parental role or not sharing information with her, which can leave her feeling isolated and replaced. It can be helpful to suggest to families that caregivers encourage children to share their sad, hurt, and angry feelings, as well as happy ones, with their mothers whenever possible. It might also be suggested that they have children request permission for activities and the like from their mother, as they did in the past, rather than consistently rely on their caregivers. Providing older siblings with a cell phone will enable them to call their mother at her bedside while they are out.

Support Systems

Families may need assistance developing support systems such as extended family, family friends, or community groups to help them during this time. Some families accustomed to giving rather than receiving help can have difficultly accepting it. May (2001) reported that they may feel a need to repay the kindness shown to them and their family, which can further add to their stress level. May also reported that coordinating this support and assistance can be challenging for some families.

Depending on their employment benefits, families may experience a decrease in family income, which can affect siblings' activities and routine. Mothers on bed rest who are employed are usually unable to continue working or will have a significant cut in their hours. Some may be required to begin their family medical leave earlier than anticipated. Their partners may also need to reduce work hours to take on additional responsibilities at home. Parents who have to hire outside help for household duties or to care for their children may see an even greater decline in their household budgets.

Families may be able to find support and assistance on bed rest issues from support groups. Maloni and Kutil (2000) reported that providing opportunities for hospitalized mothers on bed rest to get together and support one another can assist with coping in a number of areas, including family matters. McCartney (2004) described Sidelines (http://www.sidelines.org) as a helpful informative support system for mothers on bed rest. This web site has resources on a variety of topics for mothers on bed rest, including family support and resources for children.

PARENTS' TOUR OF THE NICU

A tour of the NICU can often be beneficial for families. It gives parents a first-hand look at where their new baby may be hospitalized, as well as an opportunity to discuss their questions and concerns. Griffin, Kavanaugh, Soto, and White (1997) recommended that families that have been informed that their baby may spend time in the NICU consider going on a tour before the baby is born. After interviewing a small number of parents who had received tours of the hospital during their high-risk pregnancy, they reported that the tours helped reduce parents' fears and anxieties about the hospital, made them feel more comfortable, and gave them a better understanding of the hospital environment. They also stated that information should be shared with parents about the NICU environment, the type of care their baby might receive, and the role that parents will have while their baby is in the hospital.

A tour of the hospital can provide an opportunity for families to learn about sibling issues as well. Families that may not have considered these issues in advance can benefit if the information provided by the hospital includes such topics as sibling support and visitation and unit policies regarding these issues. Rozdilsky (2005) recommended that sibling policies be discussed with all families, not just those that ask questions or request information. Families should be given copies of information and handouts during the tour so that they can read through this material before their baby is admitted.

Mr. and Mrs. Lopez visited their obstetrician for a scheduled ultrasound that showed that their baby had a diaphragmatic hernia, or a hole in his diaphragm. They were referred to a specialist who provided detailed information about how this may affect their baby's health following delivery as well as several options of ways to proceed. Both parents, who were expecting a healthy, full-term baby, were overwhelmed by the information they received. They had already begun preparing their 4-year-old daughter, Eliza, for the birth of her new baby brother but had no idea how or when to share this new information with her. They were also unsure where to go for support and assistance with this issue.

Several months before their baby was born, they were encouraged to tour the NICU where their baby would be hospitalized following birth. During the tour, they were provided with written information on sibling issues, which included how to share information with siblings. Mrs. Lopez had further questions after the tour and contacted the NICU child life specialist for further information.

WHEN THE MOTHER GOES INTO LABOR

Parents often need to be encouraged to prepare in advance for sibling issues related to the baby's birth. Some issues might include who will be available to care for siblings when parents leave for the hospital, where they will stay, and what information will be shared with them. They may also need to think about what their children will observe when their mother goes into labor. Parents tend to be very busy at this time and, in some families, can be worried about the health of the mother or the baby or both. They often have limited time to talk with and support their children as they prepare to leave for the hospital. Occasionally, problems can occur, such as the mother being in pain, bleeding, or needing to leave in an ambulance. In a few instances, children may even observe their mother giving birth, either before their parents can leave for the hospital or in route. These events can be very frightening for siblings and may influence how they will relate to the new baby.

At this stage in the arrival of a new baby, siblings may need additional information and support to help alleviate possible misconceptions or misunderstandings. Families may need varying amounts of assistance to provide this support. They may also have different comfort levels communicating relevant information to their children. Different cultures can have different beliefs about communicating difficult information to children, especially information related to pregnancy or sexual issues. Discussing parents' beliefs with them before communicating information to siblings is important. It is also important to honor and respect the family's beliefs and customs and not make the family feel as if they are inferior if their beliefs or customs are different from those of the majority of the health care team.

The Lo family, who moved to the United States several years ago, was expecting their third child. Their family included Mr. and Mrs. Lo; their 6-year-old son, Minh; 4-year-old daughter, Hung; and paternal grandparents. When Mrs. Lo went into labor, she experienced significant bleeding and was rushed to the hospital in an ambulance. When asked what information they would like to share with their children about the situation, Mr. and Mrs. Lo did not want to discuss it. After doing some research, the social worker discovered that in the Los' culture, this type of information was not shared with children. She supported the family's decision and informed them that she was available when they were ready to explain the situation to their children. She also provided additional ways to support their children in English and Vietnamese.

CONCLUSION

The addition of a new baby can be exciting, even after the pregnancy has been diagnosed as high risk. Providing opportunities for siblings to be included in various aspects of the pregnancy allows them to have a part in this important family event. It can also help them begin a special relationship with the new family member.

The Newborn
in the Hospital

A Stressful Time for Families

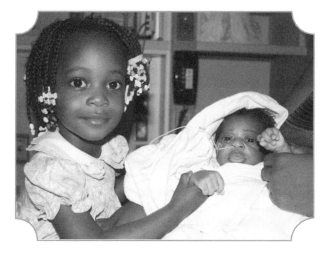

Many families feel challenged and overwhelmed when their newborn is hospitalized. Siblings may be affected not only at the time but also in the future when they revisit aspects of the hospitalization. Families often feel the loss of their ideal or imagined baby. Siblings who expected the new baby to be like those they have known or have seen on television may need assistance and support to cope with the differences between them.

When the baby is admitted to the NICU, the parental role may be interrupted or need to be adapted. For some parents, their role in the NICU can be a difficult one. They may be unable to care for their baby as they had planned or imagined during the pregnancy and may not know where to begin in this unfamiliar environment. The parental role can also be interrupted for siblings who undergo increased separation from their parents. Parents may have less involvement in some areas of their children's lives, from their daily routines to important family rituals. Parents may also be so overwhelmed by the baby's issues and various hospital experiences that they have little time and energy left for siblings.

Just as it can sometimes be difficult for parents to feel like the baby's parents when the baby is hospitalized, it can also be difficult for siblings to feel like the baby's big brother or sister. Many families often begin to prepare siblings for their role as a big brother or sister during the pregnancy. Some aspects of the sibling role may need to be adapted when the baby has been admitted to the NICU, and families may need assistance to help siblings with this adjustment.

These siblings tend to be separated from the baby more than siblings of healthy, full-term babies are. Some babies must be transferred to hospitals far from their family's home, making it difficult for siblings to visit and interact with them. Some families may not have the finances, ability, or energy to provide or encourage sibling visitation. Also, unit policies in some NICUs may limit sibling visitation to certain times or days of the week that might not fit well with siblings' regular routines. Issues such as parents' job responsibilities or lack of transportation and the cost of parking can further limit sibling visitation.

Parents are often given large amounts of verbal and written information during the first few days or weeks of the baby's admission to the NICU. Processing this amount of information, let alone explaining it to their children, can be difficult for parents. They are also coping with their own emotional issues at this time, which can make it difficult for them to assist siblings with their coping issues. Children may never have seen their parents this worried or concerned, and it can be frightening for them.

POTENTIAL DEVELOPMENTAL RESPONSES

Younger siblings can benefit from visiting their mother in the hospital, or if visits are not an option, talking with her on the telephone. They can also benefit from visiting the baby. Some families may need assistance with scheduling visits, especially around important sibling routines such as school. Because of family issues or sibling visitation guidelines or policies, it may be a few days before siblings are able to see the baby, which can be frustrating. Like their parents, siblings may want to be involved with the baby right away. In this case, it can be beneficial to give siblings a picture of the baby and suggest that they find a picture of themselves, or draw one, that can be taped to the baby's bed. They might also help choose items for the baby's bedside and hats or socks for the baby to wear.

Older siblings, too, may want to visit their mother and the baby. Some may worry about the baby's long-term prognosis and develop fears that the baby is going to die. Their personal experience with the hospital environment, especially the intensive care environment, may be limited, and their impressions of what happens there may be formed from what they have seen on television. Even though they are older, these siblings still need preparation for their visit and opportunities to voice their questions and concerns.

COPING AND PAST EXPERIENCES

Families are not always prepared for the changes in family life that a baby hospitalized in the NICU can bring, and some may require assistance to understand and adjust to these changes. Siblings can have expectations that their family life will return to normal after the baby is born, and they may become confused, frustrated, and possibly angry when this does not happen. They will often need understanding and support to adjust to the new "normal" in their family's life.

As mentioned previously, the family's prior pregnancy and birth experiences can influence how they view and cope with their current situation. Siblings who have witnessed typical pregnancy and birth experiences in their family or friends' families may expect that this experience will be similar. Their parents may believe that they will react to the birth of this baby as they have to the birth of healthy, full-term babies. Parents should take into consideration that because this pregnancy and birth is high risk, sibling issues and support may need to be adapted. Siblings who have had previous experience with the NICU may expect that this hospitalization will be identical or similar and can have difficulty if it turns out to be different. Families should be encouraged to share information with these siblings about how their current situation may differ from those they have experienced in the past.

For some families, the hospitalization of their baby in the NICU may not be the only stressful experience they are dealing with or have recently dealt with. This additional stress can affect the way family members cope and adjust. Siblings may be further affected by stressful events specific to their own lives. These may include staying with unfamiliar caregivers or being bounced from caregiver to caregiver, beginning or completing a school year, attending a new school, going to camp, or having a best friend move away. Parents should be reminded that stress can be cumulative not only for themselves, but also for siblings. They may need assistance with providing developmentally appropriate support for their children and identifying individuals to support siblings when they are not available.

SHARING INFORMATION WITH SIBLINGS

Following the baby's admission to the NICU, siblings may be with their families as they talk with physicians and other professionals. Even if they do not appear to be listening, they are often taking in not only the information being discussed, but also their parents' reactions. This situation can lead to a variety of misconceptions. Some siblings may misunderstand some of the terminology or medical jargon used to describe the baby's condition and develop a very different understanding than what was intended. Siblings also observe their parents as they begin to cope with a having a critically ill baby. Some parents become very upset and anxious and cry in front of the sibling without being able to provide explanations about why they are upset. When siblings are present but are not acknowledged as participants in these discussions, they can begin to feel invisible, ignored, or excluded.

If siblings are prohibited from participating in these conversations, they may not only feel left out of an important family event, but also begin to imagine what is being discussed behind closed doors. Some ways to include siblings in these discussions are to acknowledge their presence; provide brief, age-appropriate explanations of the information; and allow them to voice their questions and concerns. For more information about talking to siblings about the baby's hospitalization, see Chapter 4.

Tip for Families

Many NICUs have professionals such as neonatal child life specialists or neonatal social workers who are specially trained to assist families with sharing information with siblings.

SPECIAL CIRCUMSTANCES
RELATED TO THE MOTHER'S HEALTH

Many mothers of babies admitted to the NICU are discharged from the hospital a few days after giving birth. It can often be difficult for these mothers to leave their baby behind at the hospital. It can also be difficult for siblings if their mother is hospitalized longer than was expected or needs to be rehospitalized, either because of a preexisting medical condition or the diagnosis of a new medical condition. It can also be devastating for siblings and their entire family if the mother dies during or following childbirth. Should any of these events occur, there is a potential for some siblings to blame the baby. They will need frequent and developmentally appropriate explanations about their mother's condition or death to help them understand what has happened. For example, even very young siblings can understand that doctors are needed to help Mommy's heart get better or to help make Mommy breathe better.

If their mother's hospitalization has been extended, siblings can benefit from frequent contact with her, either through visits or telephone calls. It is also beneficial at this time for siblings to stay at home as often as possible rather than with relatives or friends. They are already separated from their mother and the new baby and can have difficulty if they are separated from other family members and their home environment as well. Siblings whose mother died in childbirth will experience great trauma and may benefit from programs that are available to children who have experienced the death of a parent. The social worker or child life specialist may be able to assist the family to locate these resources in their local area. Some siblings may need individualized assistance and support, which the health care team may also be able to locate for the family.

HELPING SIBLINGS COPE

The baby's admission to the NICU can affect the amount of time that parents and siblings spend together. This may be the first time they have been separated, and if the baby has been transferred to a hospital far from their home, parents and siblings may be separated even more. Parents may need gentle reminders about how important they continue to be to siblings. They may also need assistance in discovering ways to remain involved in the baby's care on a regular basis while continuing to share important routines and rituals with siblings, even if these need to be adapted.

Examples might include videotaping themselves reading the sibling's favorite bedtime stories to be played as part of the sibling's bedtime routine if they are visiting the baby during that time, eating breakfast as a family rather than dinner if they are visiting the baby after work, or helping with homework over the telephone if they are at the hospital for days at a time. Encouraging parents to maintain regular contact with siblings can help reinforce that siblings continue to be loved, are valued family members, and have not been forgotten or replaced.

Celebrating the Baby's Birth

Due to the baby's critical diagnosis and admission to the hospital, it can be difficult for families to celebrate the baby's birth as they might have if the baby had been healthy and full term. It can be especially difficult if they are unsure of the baby's diagnosis or are concerned that the baby may not survive. It can also be difficult if family members are separated.

The baby's birth is an important family event that many siblings have been anticipating for quite a while, and there are several ways to help them celebrate even though the baby is in the NICU. Siblings may want to assist in calling, e-mailing, or text-messaging family and friends to let them know the baby has arrived. Young siblings may enjoy sharing cookies, cupcakes, or special candy with friends or classmates, the way some fathers pass out cigars following the birth of a baby. They may also enjoy wearing a special big brother or sister T-shirt or button while visiting their mother or baby in the hospital.

Including Siblings in the Baby's Hospitalization

Following the baby's admission to the NICU, some families can be overwhelmed and need assistance to consider ways to involve siblings in the baby's hospitalization from the start. Providing opportunities for siblings to visit the baby allows them to see for themselves where the baby is and where their parents go when they visit the baby. Siblings may enjoy picking out a balloon or toy for the baby, creating artwork for the baby's bedside, and having their own photographs of the baby.

Some siblings may want to create a name sign with the name their family has chosen for the baby and hang it near the baby's bedside. If the family has also decided on a nickname, it should be included as well. Name signs can help siblings locate the baby's bed when they visit and can also help members of the health care team remember the baby's name and gender. It is helpful to inform families of hospital policies regarding the size of signs and how much of a patient's name can be posted at the bedside. It can be frustrating for siblings to spend time making a beautiful sign only to learn that it cannot be used.

Some families may decide to wait before allowing siblings to visit the baby in the NICU. Such decisions can be based on cultural or religious issues or previous health care experiences. These families should be supported in their decision and given alternative suggestions, such as exchanging pictures between siblings and the baby or sharing a video with siblings that includes various members of the family and health care team at the baby's bedside, as well as suggestions for literature about having a baby in the NICU to read with siblings.

Providing Opportunities to Share Concerns

Siblings can benefit from opportunities to discuss some of the issues connected with having a baby brother or sister in the NICU. These may include the baby's birth, diagnosis, and admission to the NICU, as well as separation from parents and changes in family routines and rituals. When the baby is admitted, parents may be too preoccupied to explain these issues to siblings in developmentally appropriate language. In this case, members of the baby's health care team can serve as role models for family members on the best ways to communicate with siblings as they interact with the baby. As with other issues, it is important to consider family communication and coping patterns as well as cultural issues.

Reading Books About the Hospitalization

Bibliotherapy can assist children in coping with a wide range of stressful experiences. Many families often enjoy reading books together, and reading or listening to books about aspects of the NICU experience can help facilitate conversations between siblings and the adults who care for them. Davies (2003) reported that bibliotherapy can help reduce isolation, provide opportunities for discussion, and assist with problem solving and coping. Ahmann (1997) recommended that professionals be knowledgeable about books before suggesting them to families. Families should also be provided with locations to find books, as this can sometimes be difficult for families under stress. It can be helpful to maintain a library of sibling resources for families as well (see Figure 1). (See Resources at the end of this book for suggested books.)

When deciding which books to suggest to a family, siblings' developmental and reading levels should be taken into account, and sometimes the adults' reading level as well. Book illustrations should also be considered. Manworren and Woodring (1998) reported that young children often use illustrations to help them read books to themselves, which can be beneficial when parents are busy doing other things. Preschool children tend to enjoy listening to the same book read over and over, so it can be helpful if the book is one that adults in the family enjoy as well. School-age children who are learning to read can still benefit from having stories read to them.

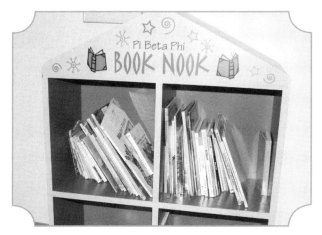

Figure 1.   NICUs can maintain a library of sibling resources for families to share.

Another issue to consider is the accuracy of the text and illustrations. It should also be noted how closely this information matches the policies and procedures of the particular institution, as well as the sibling's and family's specific experiences. The family's cultural and religious beliefs should be considered, too, as families may be reluctant to use books that infringe on their beliefs.

Siblings should be given a choice about participating in this activity. Cohen (1987) reported that children should not be forced to read or listen to a specific story, but should be given choices. They will be ready for this activity at different times, and some children may never want to participate.

CONCLUSION

In some homes, family life may temporarily stop due to the focus on the baby's problems and admission to the NICU. However, if the baby is hospitalized for an extended time, siblings should not have to put their needs on hold for the duration. Extracurricular activities, play dates, planned activities with parents, and summer plans may be canceled, postponed, or changed, which can be difficult for siblings to cope with. Meeting the needs of all their children can be difficult for families with a baby in the NICU. Therefore, they may benefit from suggested ways to meet siblings' needs.

Talking with Big Brothers and Sisters

What Do We Tell Them?

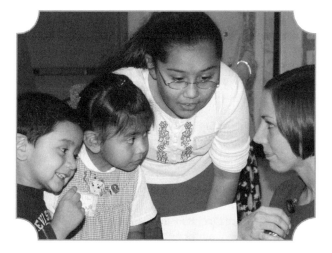

Some families may be reluctant to discuss issues concerning the baby's hospitalization with their children. Parents report how difficult the information is for adults in the family to understand and cope with, so how can they expect their children to handle it? They may also want to protect or shield siblings from what they perceive as difficult information and emotions, or they believe that their children are too young to understand these issues. Some may decide to wait until the baby has a definite diagnosis or siblings begin to ask questions. Others may want to talk with their children but have difficulty putting the information into developmentally appropriate language, so they end up saying nothing at all. Parents who are separated from their children due to the distance of the hospital from the family's home may not feel comfortable discussing issues over the telephone or having caregivers share information with their children. Some families may refuse to discuss various issues with siblings for cultural or religious reasons, or because of negative experiences with health care in the past. These decisions should be respected without making the family feel guilty.

WITHHOLDING INFORMATION FROM SIBLINGS

Information that is shared with siblings about the hospitalization of the baby can affect how they perceive the situation as well as how they cope with it. Peebles-Kleiger (2000) reported that not sharing information with children can reduce their ability to receive the support they need and can affect the ways they cope and adjust. Sometimes siblings get information that their families did not intend for them to hear from adult conversations and telephone calls they have overheard. When information is not shared with siblings directly, there is a risk that these conversations will be the only information they receive. Siblings may also use their imagination to fill in any gaps, which can lead to further misunderstandings and misconceptions. If the baby or the baby's hospitalization are topics avoided in family conversations, siblings can feel alone with their thoughts and feelings. They may blame themselves by believing that they have somehow caused the baby's hospitalization or diagnosis or their parents' increased emotional distress.

Charlie, who was 4, wished that his mother had never become pregnant because there was not enough room on her lap to snuggle. His 6-year-old sister, Tamara, thought it would be nice if the baby went home with another family because she heard from a friend at school that all babies do is cry all the time. If their mother comes home from the hospital no longer pregnant and without the baby, these siblings may believe that their thoughts and wishes came true, particularly if they are not provided with explanations in developmentally appropriate language.

Three-year-old Shaniqua accidentally kicked her mother's tummy as her mother was helping her dress one morning, and every night as her mother puts her 5-year-old brother, Leo, to bed, he asks, "When are you going to come out, baby?" Several days later, their mother went into premature labor, and a week later, the baby died. These siblings may believe that their actions or words caused their mother's premature labor and the baby's death, especially if they are not given explanations that they are able to understand.

Juan noticed that since his baby sister was born and admitted to the hospital, his papá didn't have time to play catch with him anymore. His papá was usually at work, and when he was home, he was always on the telephone or working at the computer. Juan thought his papá didn't want to play with him and that he loved the baby more than he loved him, because he accidentally broke Papá's favorite coffee cup. He does not understand that his father is working overtime to help pay the baby's medical bills and that he is struggling to keep up with the insurance paperwork.

Three big sisters, ages 7, 9, and 10, were very excited when their baby brother was born. Their parents explained that he was born early and needed to stay in the hospital a while, but they did not provide any additional information as his hospitalization progressed. Several weeks later, the baby began to show signs of necrotizing entercolitis (NEC). The parents were very concerned but continued to not share information with their daughters. The girls were aware of their parents growing distress but did not know the reason for it. They began to have difficulty sleeping and completing their schoolwork and argued more. They overheard their parents discussing NEC, and thought that one of their parents had cancer in their neck and was going to die of cancer like their grandfather had several years ago.

DISCUSSING THE BABY'S HOSPITALIZATION

When discussing the baby's hospitalization with siblings, their developmental level should be considered. Issues such as learning differences and developmental delays can also influence their perception of the situation, as well as their ability to understand and process information. Hansdottir and Malcarne (1998) and Myant and Williams (2005) reported that as children grow and mature, their understanding of illness issues tends to grow and mature as well. Young children, however, can sometimes understand aspects of complex illness issues. Raman and Gelman (2005) stated that young children have the ability to understand some of the differences between the spread of illness in genetic and contagious conditions.

Older Infant Siblings

Older infants are not able to cognitively understand what is happening in the NICU, but they are able to sense changes in stress levels and routines in their home environment. Deering and Cody (2002) discussed that eye contact and gentle vocal tones, as well as comfort and reassurance, are effective ways to communicate with infants. They also mentioned the importance of being aware of overstimulation cues when interacting with them. The NICU waiting room and hospital environment, as well as the environment of other caregivers, may not only be overstimulating for infant siblings, but may also be a significant change from their regular daily routine.

Toddler Siblings

With toddlers, explanations about the baby should be brief and simple and take into account their short attention span. It can also be beneficial to relate the baby's diagnosis to an external body part to help facilitate their understanding. This can be much easier for some diagnoses than for others. For example, a myelomeningocele might be described as "a boo-boo on the baby's back" or a gastroschisis might be described as "an ouchie on the baby's tummy." Some diagnoses, such as congenital heart disease and respiratory distress, can be more difficult to describe in this manner. In these situations, it may be beneficial to point to the baby's or toddler's chest and show them where the baby needs special help. MacWhinney, Cermak, and Fisher (1987) reported a significant increase in the ability of children to identify external body parts at around 2 years of age. Toddlers are egocentric and focus primarily on their own needs, which should also be considered when providing them with information.

Preschool Siblings

Preschoolers tend to interpret information literally, which can lead to numerous misunderstandings and misconceptions. Medical jargon, unfamiliar to most preschoolers, can easily be misinterpreted. Table 1 shows examples of medical jargon typically misunderstood by young siblings, the possible misunderstanding, and examples of developmentally appropriate explanations. Jensen (1995) mentioned that children can repeat words without understanding their complete meaning. Preschoolers can sometimes appear to have an accurate understanding of issues when, in fact, they are just parroting the words they have heard. Explanations should be expressed in terms that preschool siblings can easily understand and in a format that provides opportunities for further discussion.

Table 1. Medical jargon often misunderstood by young siblings

Medical jargon	Misunderstanding	Explanation
N-I-C-U "Nic-u"	I see you? Nick who?	The neonatal intensive care unit is a special place in the hospital for brand new babies who need some extra help after they are born. It is a long name, so it is sometimes shortened to NICU or Nic-u.
27 weeker	Is the baby getting weaker?	When babies are born early, we count how many weeks they were inside their mother before they were born. Your baby was inside your mom for 27 weeks before he was born, so we sometimes call him a 27 weeker. This does not mean that he is getting weaker. In fact, we expect him to get stronger every day.
Urine	You're in what?	Urine is a word we use for pee, like going to the bathroom. What word do you use?
Urinate	The baby's not 8 years old. (You're an/in eight.)	Urinate is a word we use for going to the bathroom. What word do you use?
Stool	Do you have a special baby stool or seat for the baby to sit on?	Stool is a word we use for poop, like going to the bathroom. What word do you use?
IV	Why does the baby need to have a plant growing out of her body? (Ivy)	The IV is a way for the baby to get medicine and other important things. IV is short for a very long word, intravenous. It is important to keep it there because the baby needs the medicine to get better.
Draw blood	Why are you going to draw a picture with the baby's blood?	We are going to draw or take a tiny amount of the baby's blood to help us better understand what is happening inside the baby's body and to make sure that the baby is getting the right amount of medicine.
Arterial line	Is the baby going to do art? (Art line)	An arterial line is a way for us to see if the baby is getting enough oxygen.
CAT scan	Is there a cat in there?	A CAT scan is one way to take a picture of the inside of the baby's body from the outside. There are no cats in a CAT scan.
Dye	Is my baby going to die?	Dye is a colored liquid, like colored water, that helps us learn more about the inside of the baby's body.
NEC	What is the matter with the baby's neck?	NEC is short for necrotizing enterocolitis. NEC is a problem with the baby's insides, or intestines. They are not working the way they should be. Do you want to see where the intestines are on this drawing?
Grade I IVH	The baby's not in the first grade. I'm in kindergarten, and I'm bigger than the baby. (Grade one)	This is one of the ways we keep track of how the baby's brain is doing.

School-Age Siblings

School-age children can understand more detailed information about the baby, and some often have a variety of questions and concerns. Rozdilsky (2005) discussed that school-age children have a better ability to comprehend than they do to share, so rather than wait for them to ask questions, they should be asked whether they would like additional information. In addition, reflective listening and an awareness of their body language can also help provide insight into school-age siblings' understanding of the information and their emotions. Explanations should be phrased clearly, as these siblings also frequently misinterpret medical jargon and terminology.

Preteen and Adolescent Siblings

Preteens and adolescents usually have had little experience with health care issues, especially those related to pregnancy, newborns, and intensive care. Their ability to understand medical jargon and terminology in these areas can be limited as well. They might also equate the baby's NICU experience to something similar they have seen on television medical shows, often a primary source of medical information for preteens and adolescents. They often appreciate being asked for input, ideas, and suggestions but may be reluctant to share them for fear of appearing unintelligent. All of these factors should be taken into account when explaining the baby's hospitalization to preteen and adolescent siblings.

Information Sharing and Siblings' Comprehension

Information shared with siblings should not only be developmentally appropriate but also provided in amounts siblings are able to comprehend. Too little information can leave out important details, whereas too much can overwhelm or confuse them. The amount of information siblings are ready for can be influenced by their developmental level as well as their questions and concerns.

It is helpful to talk with siblings on their schedule and at their pace. At various times they may be full of questions, have just a few questions, or have no questions at all. They may also ask the same questions repeatedly as they try to understand and process the information. Considering that they have

Tip for Families

Sharing information with siblings has the potential to help them feel included in the baby's NICU hospitalization.

fewer life experiences to draw on, shorter attention spans, and fewer coping mechanisms than adults have, it will be difficult for siblings to comprehend all of the information about the baby at one time.

Providing Truthful and Accurate Information

Another consideration for families when discussing issues with siblings is providing honest and accurate information. Williams and Binnie (2002) suggested that accurate information about illness-related issues as well as opportunities to discuss them can help increase children's understanding. Just as parents and other family members tend to appreciate individuals who are open and honest, so do siblings. This approach can also help alleviate misinterpretations and misunderstandings, as well as siblings' feelings that they may have caused the baby's hospitalization and other related problems. This can help siblings begin to acknowledge their families as an important resource for information. Families whose cultural beliefs discourage sharing difficult information with children should be informed of the importance of accurate information but supported in whatever decision they make.

Tip for Families

Telling siblings, "I don't know, but I'll find out," can provide parents with time to locate accurate responses to siblings' questions or to put difficult information into developmentally appropriate language.

Providing an Atmosphere for Open Discussion

Maintaining a receptive atmosphere can help siblings feel more comfortable asking questions and expressing concerns. Siblings should be assured that whatever their questions or concerns are, they will be accepted and appreciated. This may also help siblings feel more comfortable initiating conversations about the baby's hospitalization and related matters. Maintaining consistent eye contact while speaking to siblings is also important and can be achieved by adults squatting beside the child or bringing the child up to the adult's level. It should be noted that eye contact might not be appropriate for siblings from some cultural backgrounds.

Information Sharing as an Ongoing Process

Sharing information with siblings is an ongoing process rather than a one-time event. It should continue throughout the baby's hospitalization and after the baby is home. Like other family members, siblings need time and numerous conversations to help them process information. As they mature, their ability to process information improves, and they will probably have different and additional questions and concerns long after the baby's NICU experience is over.

Discussing Emotions

Siblings often experience a variety of emotions when the baby is hospitalized. Their comfort level in sharing them depends on issues such as their developmental level, temperament, culture, and coping abilities. Utilizing reflective listening as well as siblings' verbal and nonverbal communication can sometimes help families learn how siblings feel about this experience. Depending on the sibling's developmental level, it may also be helpful for family members to share their own feelings with siblings, bearing in mind that some of these emotions can be overwhelming for them. Children should not be made to feel they are the keeper of their parents' or other adult family members' feelings.

Assisting Siblings in Sharing Information With Others

Siblings often need assistance communicating information about the baby's experience to others, such as their friends and classmates. If their parents are spending a great deal of time away from home to accommodate the baby's hospitalization, siblings can be the family member that friends and other people in the community see on a regular basis, either in the neighborhood or at school. They may be asked repeatedly about the baby, and possibly their parents, and not know what to say.

To assist these siblings, families could develop a script for them to repeat when they are asked about the baby, perhaps practicing the script with an extended family member beforehand. They could also include it in the greeting on their family's answering machine, updating the script as the baby's condition changes. Dokken and Sydnor-Greenberg (1998) stated that updated messages on the family's answering machine can reduce the number of times they are asked about the baby's progress. Some families may not feel comfortable with this option because they are unable to control who receives the information. Another option might be a mass e-mailing, which gives families greater control over who receives information. Older siblings might assist parents in sending the e-mail, and some may want to include individuals they wish to receive it as well.

PROFESSIONAL SUPPORT AND ASSISTANCE

A variety of families may request assistance in sharing information with their children, so it can be beneficial to anticipate some of their questions and concerns. Different issues such as individual parenting styles and past NICU experiences, as well as coping, religious, and cultural issues, can influence what they will ask or want to discuss. These issues may also greatly influence what and when families are comfortable communicating information to siblings.

Parents should be supported as providers of information to their children. When their baby is admitted to the NICU, many parents can easily feel overwhelmed and inadequate in their role as parents. These feelings can intensify when parents are unsure of how to share information with their children, and they will often need help. Parents may also need support in coping with family members or health care staff who do not agree with or understand their decisions about sharing or not sharing certain information with their children.

Families may need assistance in locating appropriate health care staff to help them share information with siblings. Various members of the health care team, such as neonatal child life specialists, neonatal social workers, bedside nurses, psychologists, or psychiatrists, are often available in many NICUs to assist families. The siblings' pediatrician may also be helpful, especially if the pediatrician has had an ongoing relationship with the sibling and family, or if a sibling is being treated for the same or a similar diagnosis as the baby. Family support groups may also be a resource for information and support.

CONCLUSION

For many families, sharing information about the baby's progress in the NICU with their children is difficult. Parents should be encouraged to consider their children's developmental level, provide accurate information, and share information throughout the baby's hospitalization and after the baby is home. Families may also need assistance and support when others do not agree with their decision to share or not to share certain information with their children.

5

When Parents
Visit the Baby

Ways to Support Big Brothers and Sisters

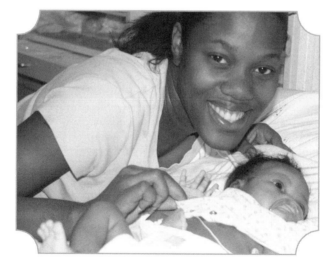

Babies who need specialized care may be transferred to a hospital far from their family's home. In a few families, mothers may go into premature labor or have other difficulties while traveling, and their babies may be hospitalized far from home as well. Fry, Cartwright, Huang, and Davies (2003) reported that parents whose babies were born while their mothers were traveling experienced financial problems, loneliness, isolation, and lack of family support. Yantzi, Rosenberg, Burke, and Harrison (2001) discussed that distance can increase the challenges and concerns that families may have, as well as affect family relationships.

The distance between the family's home and the hospital can affect the family's visitation. Transportation costs such as gas, maintenance, and parking can be prohibitive for many families or put a significant dent in the family budget. Some families may not own or have access to a vehicle and must depend on others for transportation, whereas other families may have to use public transportation, which can be time consuming and may be available only at certain times. Parents whose traveling time is considerable may decide to visit less frequently and spend longer periods visiting the baby in an effort to reduce travel time and costs, which can extend the length of time that siblings and parents are separated. Parents may need assistance and support to learn how to stay connected with and support siblings while they are visiting the baby in the NICU for extended periods.

OPPORTUNITIES FOR SIBLING VISITS WITH PARENTS

When parents are away from siblings for long periods, they should be encouraged to create opportunities for siblings to visit them. During these visits, families can enjoy reconnecting and spending time together. If they are out of town, parents can often benefit from information on inexpensive child-friendly activities located near the hospital or in the city. This information may be available on the Internet as well as other locations (e.g., local newspapers, libraries, bookstores), but many parents may be too preoccupied with the new baby to seek it out on their own. Rozdilsky (2005) suggested that these families can benefit from staying at family-friendly locations, where they may have opportunities to interact with other families of hospitalized children who may also have siblings. She also recommended creating a child-friendly atmosphere in the hospital to welcome siblings. For example, a corner of the NICU family waiting area might be designated for siblings to help them feel welcome and comfortable in an unfamiliar environment.

FAMILIAR CAREGIVERS AND ENVIRONMENTS

When parents visit the baby frequently and for extended intervals, siblings are often left without their primary support system—their parents—during a time of stress. Utilizing familiar, consistent caregivers while parents are away can

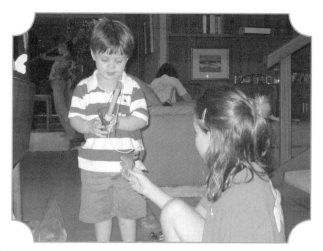

Figure 2. Siblings are a unique support system for each other if they are together.

help provide siblings with assistance and support and may also lower parents' stress. If parents are less worried about their children back home, they may be better able to focus on bonding with the baby and learning the baby's care.

Siblings, too, can be a familiar source of support for one another. If there is more than one older sibling, some families may be tempted to separate them among different extended family members or family friends as a way to reduce the amount of help they request from any one individual or family. However, siblings who are separated this way are actually being separated from a unique support system—each other (see Figure 2). Although siblings may cope differently with the baby's hospitalization, they can often be a wonderful support system for each other just by being together. The amount of support they provide will depend on their developmental level, temperament, past experiences, and the support they are receiving from other sources, such as the adults in their environment.

Siblings also tend to benefit from being able to stay in their home environment. If they must stay elsewhere, and especially if they have to be shuttled from place to place, they may not be able to sleep as well as they do in their own bed and in their own room. Some families may have limited options regarding a safe place for siblings to stay while they are with the baby in the NICU. The sibling's pillow and perhaps sheets from home can help make a different bed feel and smell more like home and possibly make bedtime less stressful. Security items such as special toys, blankets, or dolls can also be beneficial.

SUPPORTING SIBLINGS WHEN PARENTS VISIT THE BABY

Some siblings can have a difficult time watching their parents leave to visit the baby. Their parents may try to sneak away to prevent or reduce crying and distress. As a result, siblings may feel a need to be on guard for possible future disappearances. They may become more clingy and feel compelled to stay close to their parents, or at least keep them within eyesight. This can become exhausting and can greatly increase the uncertainty of the situation for them. Parents should be encouraged to let siblings know when they are leaving.

As Mrs. Katz was about to leave to visit her baby in the NICU, she sent her 3- and 5-year-old daughters to the kitchen to help their grandmother make cookies and then sneaked out the door. Minutes later, the girls ran out of the kitchen with cookies to share with their mother, only to discover that she had disappeared. They began to cry, and it took their grandmother some time to console them. When Mrs. Katz returned several hours later, the girls became very clingy and were reluctant to leave her side. They followed her from room to room and at bedtime did not want her to leave their room. They got out of bed frequently to check to make sure she had not disappeared again.

Mr. and Mrs. Hao were ready to leave to visit their baby. They went into the family room where their 6-year-old son, Lee, was watching television with his 19-year-old step-brother, Kim, and informed them that they were leaving. Lee began to cry and cling to their parents. His mother informed him that they would return just before supper and asked him to finish watching the movie with Kim so that he could tell them what happened when they got home. After Mr. and Mrs. Hao left, Lee continued to cry for a while but was easily redirected by Kim to finish watching the movie before his parents returned. Lee happily greeted his parents when they arrived home and was eager to share his favorite parts of the movie.

Andrew was dropped off with a familiar baby sitter so that his mother could visit the baby. His mother talked to Andrew's baby sitter about the baby's progress for several minutes before she left. Right before she walked out the door, she sought out Andrew to inform him that she was leaving and would return during his favorite cartoon show. Andrew began to cry but was quickly consoled by the baby sitter and easily redirected back to his play.

Siblings can also benefit from having something of their parents' to hold or take care of until they return, which will help remind them of their parents while they are gone. These items should be safe for the sibling's age and developmental level and be easily replaceable in case they become lost or damaged.

Three-year-old Lucy and 4-year-old Marc had difficulty when their parents left to visit the baby, so their mother gave Lucy an old purse to fill with special things while they were gone and gave Marc one of his dad's old T-shirts to wear until they returned.

Six-year-old Larry was anxious when his father left to visit the baby, so his father gave Larry an old set of car keys to keep until he returned, which he could jingle in his pocket just like Dad does.

Ten-year-old David and 12-year-old Danielle had difficulty when their parents left to visit the baby for several days at a time. Their parents gave them copies of important family photographs for David to tuck in his backpack and Danielle to put in her purse so that they could look at them as needed until their parents returned.

Young siblings have difficulty with the concept of time, so even when parents spend just a short time at the hospital, it can seem like an eternity to them. When parents leave, these siblings should be reassured about when their parents will return. It can be helpful to tie their parents' anticipated return into a part of the siblings' regular routines, such as after school, before dinner, after bedtime, or after a favorite TV show. If parents will be away for several days, siblings might be given a calendar so they can mark off or place a sticker on each day until their parents' return. They might also enjoy small, inexpensive wrapped surprises to open each day to mark the days until their parents are home.

Maintaining Contact with Parents

When parents are away from home for extended periods, siblings can benefit from regular contact, such as through telephone calls. Establishing a regular time to call, perhaps at bedtime or first thing each morning, will not only let siblings know when to expect the call, but also that they have not been forgotten. Parents should be reminded that toddler and preschool siblings have short attention spans, especially when they are unable to see the person they are talking to. Also, because talking on the telephone with their parents may be a new experience for some, they may have trouble understanding that it is their parents on the other end of the line. Parents should also be advised that siblings may be more interested in telling their parents what has been happening in their own lives than in hearing about the baby or what is happening at the hospital.

Another way for parents to maintain regular contact with siblings is by mail and e-mail, which many siblings especially enjoy when it is addressed to them. Some parents may need help locating mailboxes within the hospital as well as the nearest post office for stamps and other supplies. They may also need help finding where they can safely plug in their laptops or where computers with e-mail access are located for family use. If families do not have access to e-mail at home, siblings might try e-mailing from the local public library, from their school, or from a friend's or extended family member's home computer. Some hospitals also have e-mail sites for family and friends to send e-mails to patients. This can be useful if siblings want to send messages back to their parents and to the baby. Providing disposable cameras for families who do not have their own might also be considered. Parents who are reluctant to leave the baby's bedside will particularly benefit from assistance in these areas.

Supporting Toddler and Preschool Siblings

For toddler and preschool siblings, being separated from their parents is often one of the most difficult aspects of having a new baby hospitalized in the NICU. This may be the first time siblings have been separated from their parents this frequently or even overnight. Although toddler and preschool siblings may understand that their parents are at the hospital to see the baby, they can have difficulty visualizing the hospital and what their parents are doing there.

Pictures of various places in the hospital, such as the baby's bed space or where their parents wait to see the baby, and of the friendly faces of the special people who help care for the baby can give siblings an idea of what the hospital is like before they visit. These pictures, along with explanations about them, can also help reduce some of the misconceptions and misunderstandings siblings may have. Some examples of these misconceptions might include Mommy, Daddy, and the baby are having a great time without me; the baby is having a party, and I'm not invited; the baby is getting lots of presents; the people at the hospital are scary and are hurting my baby; the baby is scared because he is all by himself; they don't feed the babies at the hospital; or my baby is really dead. Pictures can be kept in a sturdy photo album for easy access and to enable siblings to share them with caregivers, friends, and family.

Whether toddler and preschool siblings are cared for in their own home or are staying somewhere else while their parents are visiting the baby, safety issues should be considered. Of special concern is siblings' access to caregivers' medication, especially when siblings are being cared for by their grandparents or other older relatives or friends. The Minnesota Poison Control System (2004) reported that these individuals may be taking numerous medications that young children can find in purses and overnight bags of older adults visiting their home. It also mentioned the need to keep other medications and dangerous substances out of the child's reach. Adult caregivers without children in their own home on a regular basis may not think about placing medication out of siblings' reach, may be less likely to use child-resistant packaging, or may leave tops off containers because they are difficult to open.

Supporting School-Age and Preteen Siblings

School-age and preteen siblings have a better understanding of the hospital environment than younger siblings do, although (as stated previously) much of what they know may come from what they have seen on television or learned from their friends. These siblings can benefit from opportunities to contact their parents, especially when they need to discuss important issues and only Mom or Dad will do. Like younger siblings, they may also enjoy having photographs of the baby and of their parents with the baby, which they can keep in an album with space for additional photographs as the baby continues to grow and develop, and which they can share with others.

RECONNECTING AS A
FAMILY BETWEEN PARENTAL VISITS

When parents return home from visiting the baby, they may get caught up in all the chores that may have been put on hold while they were gone, such as cooking, cleaning, laundry, and errands. Also, some parents may be working overtime to reduce the amount of vacation time they may be using when they visit the baby or to help with extra expenses, leaving them even less time to spend with siblings.

It is important for family members to reconnect as a family unit between parents' extended visits to the hospital, either by eating meals together, playing together, or joining together in favorite activities. Parents should seek opportunities to reconnect with siblings individually on a regular basis, such as going for walks, playing sports, going out to eat, or doing crafts or hobbies together.

When families reconnect between parental visits to the NICU, it provides opportunities for parents to help continue with family routines and

---

Tip for Families

Consider how often family time and siblings' time with parents are interrupted by the telephone or the computer. It may be beneficial to turn off the cell phone, let the answering machine answer the telephone, and shut down the computer during this time.

rituals. It also provides opportunities for them to introduce the baby into some of the sibling's daily routines at home, which may help siblings begin to perceive the baby as an important member of the family. Some ways to introduce the baby through routines might be adding the baby's pictures to family pictures around the house; talking about the baby throughout the day, such as what the baby might be doing at that particular time; or praying for the baby during siblings' bedtime prayers or family prayer time.

CONCLUSION

When a baby is hospitalized in the NICU, many parents will visit the baby without their other children. During these visits, they often bond with their new baby, learn about their baby's medical issues, participate in the baby's routine care, and learn some of the baby's specialized care needs. These visits may be extended, especially if the hospital is located a great distance from the family's home. Parents should be encouraged to support siblings by providing familiar caregivers and environments, as well as maintaining regular contact and reconnecting as a family when they return—especially if they are away for extended periods of time. Other ways parents can assist siblings when they visit the baby include informing siblings when they are leaving, tying their return into a part of the sibling's daily routine, and providing pictures to help reduce siblings' misunderstandings about what their parents and the baby are doing together without them.

6

Big Brothers and Sisters Visit the Baby

How to Make It a Success

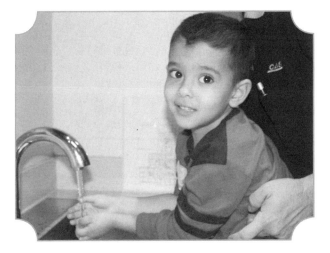

Many siblings are interested in visiting the baby in the NICU, and, if they are unable to do so, they can feel excluded from this important family event. Visiting, talking to, and touching the baby allows siblings to begin the bonding process or to continue the process begun during the mother's pregnancy. Visitations also help siblings begin to integrate the baby into their family, as well as recognize the baby as a separate and unique individual with his or her own set of needs, likes, and dislikes.

The American Academy of Pediatrics (1985) reported that sibling visitation is an important aspect of family-centered care. As policies and procedures are developed, it is important to include siblings in the unit's and hospital's definition of family-centered care. Staff can have a variety of issues or concerns about siblings visiting in the NICU. Meyer, Kennally, Zika-Beres, Cashore, and Oh (1996) reported that NICU staff's concerns decreased and sibling visitation was viewed more positively after a sibling visitation program had been put in place. Staff can also help make sibling visitation programs successful. Montgomery, Kleiber, Nicholson, and Craft-Rosenberg (1997) described a sibling visitation approach in the NICU that had been adapted by nursing staff to make the process less time consuming and easier to follow. They described how materials were arranged and were made easily accessible to staff when they were needed.

BENEFITS OF SIBLING VISITS

Sibling visitations can provide valuable information to the baby's bedside caregivers. Occasionally during sibling visits, the health care team can become aware of safety concerns, siblings' developmental delays, or health issues that need to be addressed before the baby goes home. It is much easier to address these issues early in the baby's hospitalization rather than later in the discharge process or after the baby is home.

Several studies have reported that visiting the baby in the hospital can be a positive experience for siblings. Schwab, Tolbert, Bagnato, and Maisels (1983) reported that siblings who visited the baby in the NICU described the hospital in more positive ways, had reduced fantasies and misconceptions about the NICU and the baby, and felt more included in this important family event. Ballard, Maloney, Shank, and Hollister (1984) reported that siblings' responses were positive but varied with their developmental level, with younger siblings more interested in the NICU environment and older siblings more interested in the baby. Oehler and Vileisis (1990) reported that siblings who visited the baby in the NICU demonstrated fewer negative behaviors and a greater knowledge about the baby and the baby's issues than siblings who did not visit.

Some babies may be hospitalized for extended periods, which can make it more difficult for siblings and other family members to bond and interact with them. The relationship between siblings is important, and providing opportunities to get it off to a positive start while the baby is in the hospital is beneficial. Ways in which siblings respond to visiting the baby in the NICU often depend on their developmental level, although siblings at the same developmental level may respond differently on the basis of their temperaments, past experiences, support systems, and coping abilities.

Tip for Families

Siblings in the same family can focus on different issues in the NICU or cope differently, even if they are close in age. Also, the same sibling can have different reactions during different visits to the NICU.

Sibling visits can benefit the baby as well. They give the baby an opportunity to not only interact with his or her siblings, but also to begin the bonding process with his or her family as a unit. In addition, sibling visitations and interactions with family members can offer the baby a sense of familiarity that can help the baby adapt to the home environment.

TODDLER SIBLINGS

Providing opportunities for toddler siblings to visit the baby gives them a chance to begin to learn ways to interact safely and appropriately with the new baby and also gives the family time to bond and interact. Toddlers can have difficulty comprehending exactly what has happened. They may be aware that the baby is no longer in Mommy's tummy, but without support and developmentally appropriate explanations, they may be unsure of where the baby is now. It can also be difficult for them to understand that the baby is in the hospital if they are unable to actually see the baby there.

Their visits with the baby can help reassure them where the baby is and can provide a reference for future conversations about the baby. For example, parents can say, "Remember, the baby is in the hospital. We went to see him there. You gave him the balloon, and he gave you the big sister T-shirt. Here is the picture that the nurse took of us while we were there." Also, because toddlers tend to have short attention spans and are easily distracted, their visits should be kept brief.

PRESCHOOL SIBLINGS

Visiting the baby in the NICU can provide the visual reference that many preschoolers may need to help clarify and reduce possible misconceptions and misunderstandings. Their perception of the hospital and the NICU may be some faraway place the baby has been sent for some unknown reason. Meeting various members of the health care team can help reassure them that someone is taking good care of the baby when they or their parents are not around. During their visits, preschool siblings can also learn how to interact safely with the baby and how to assist with the baby's care.

Tip for Families

Siblings can enjoy bringing a special gift for the baby, especially during their first visit. Some examples might be a small stuffed animal, a toy, or a balloon.

SCHOOL-AGE SIBLINGS

During visits to the baby in the hospital, school-age siblings can learn how to interact safely and help provide care without overstimulating the baby. Andrade (1998) stated that sibling visitation provides opportunities for bedside caregivers to share information with siblings about the baby. These members of the health care team may be able to help clarify some of the misconceptions and misunderstandings siblings may have about the baby's issues. Visiting the NICU also gives siblings a chance to meet and begin to develop a relationship with consistent members of the baby's health care team.

PRETEEN SIBLINGS

Visiting the baby in the NICU can help preteen siblings learn more about the baby's hospital experience and medical condition. Preteen siblings can also learn ways to interact with the baby and participate in the baby's care from consistent members of the baby's health care team. As they become more familiar with these caregivers, they may feel more comfortable about asking them for information.

ADOLESCENT SIBLINGS

Adolescent siblings may be interested in learning aspects of the baby's care during their visits, but may have little experience with infants and can be apprehensive. Some adolescents may hesitate to share all their questions and concerns with family members for a variety of reasons, so developing a relationship with members of the baby's health care team can be beneficial for them.

SCHEDULING SIBLING VISITS

The timing of sibling visits should be a family decision and can be based on issues such as siblings' interest level, parents' preference, the family's cultural beliefs, siblings' developmental level, distance between the hospital and home, and the family's available transportation. In some NICUs, sibling visitation guidelines and policies can also affect the timing of sibling visits. Other matters to consider when planning for sibling visits are the health of the baby, the mother, and the siblings. If the mother has health problems following delivery, families may have difficulty providing transportation and support for siblings. Also, visits will need to be postponed or rescheduled if siblings are sick or have been exposed to an illness.

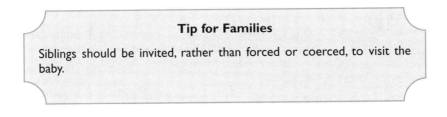

Tip for Families

Siblings should be invited, rather than forced or coerced, to visit the baby.

Frequency and Length of Visits

The frequency and length of sibling visits can vary from sibling to sibling. Some siblings may want to visit often, some not at all, and others may be somewhere in between. Also, some siblings may want to have long visits in order to interact with and help care for the baby, whereas others may just want to check in and see how the baby is doing. The frequency and length of visits can be affected by siblings' developmental level, temperament, interest, and attention span, as well as the baby's health and any procedures that may be occurring at the baby's bedside. The length of visits can also vary as siblings' interest levels change throughout the baby's hospitalization. Allowing siblings to have choices about the frequency and length of their visits gives them some control over how their relationship with the baby develops, which can help them cope with this experience.

Sibling Routines

Some families may need assistance deciding when to schedule sibling visits. The baby's caregiving needs, such as their sleep and feeding schedule, as well as any scheduled procedures should be considered along with siblings' daily routines. Younger siblings may have difficulty focusing on the baby when they are tired and hungry and can be easily overwhelmed and prone to temper tantrums. Therefore, planning visits around their naptimes and mealtimes may be beneficial. Older siblings are usually involved in school and extracurricular activities, as well as in activities with their friends. These activities should be kept as consistent and predictable as possible, with visits scheduled around them. If they have to miss school consistently to visit the baby, they can fall behind, and some schools may be reluctant to excuse siblings on a regular basis. Siblings may also become frustrated or resentful if they are consistently forced to choose between visiting the baby and participating in an activity they enjoy.

Travel Time

Parents who must travel a great distance to and from the hospital and are already under stress may have limited tolerance for exuberant siblings who accompany them. They can become upset with siblings who do not sit still and stay quiet on the way to the hospital, during the visit with the baby, and on the way home. Staying quiet and still for extended periods is often difficult for children, especially younger children who tend to have short attention spans, and this can influence how often parents are willing to take siblings with them to visit the baby.

Some hospitals have sibling activity rooms that can help families with this issue. Siblings are able to release some of their pent-up energy before they visit the baby in the NICU and again before the ride home. If this option is not available, families should be provided with information on inexpensive child-friendly activities, such as playgrounds or activity centers, located near the hospital.

Bedside caregivers may want to consider having special activities available in case siblings become restless and need a break while visiting at the baby's bedside. These activities may include coloring pictures or going with the bedside caregiver to gather clean linen or other supplies for the baby. Families may also need suggestions for travel activities. These activities should be safe and developmentally appropriate as well as inexpensive. In some hospitals, the volunteer services department may be able to help by providing families with toys that have been donated to the hospital. If parents remain reluctant to take siblings along to visit the baby, it might be suggested that they take videos and photographs of the baby to share with siblings at home.

STAFF AND FAMILY PREPARATION

Among the issues that should be considered before sibling visitations are the hospital sibling visitation policies and guidelines. These can vary from hospital to hospital, and families should be given a copy of this information. Some hospitals allow siblings to visit only on certain days or at certain times. Siblings can become upset if they are expecting to visit the baby on a specific day and then learn that they have to wait due to a hospital policy.

Families can also become frustrated if they perceive that some members of the baby's caregiving team are willing to bend the rules but others are not. Many families are better able to understand why and when rules can and cannot be bent when explanations are provided.

Tip for Families

Ask for copies of sibling visitation policies and guidelines.

Important Locations

Young siblings can quickly become hungry, thirsty, or in need of a potty and may have difficulty waiting for an adult to find the cafeteria or a restroom. Knowing where various places are in the hospital can help facilitate sibling visits and reduce some of this waiting time. Examples of these areas might be

- Waiting room
- Nearest restroom and water fountain
- Desk where siblings check in
- Sinks where siblings can wash their hands
- Support services for siblings of NICU patients (Sometimes these services, such as a sibling program for the entire hospital, are located in another area of the hospital.)
- Closest snack and drink machines
- Hospital cafeteria and other places that provide food or snacks, especially places that are child friendly

The path siblings should take through the NICU to get to the baby's bedside is also important. Families and the health care team need to be aware of what siblings might observe as they pass by other babies' bedsides.

Distractions at the Baby's Bedside

Limiting the number of visitors and reducing distractions around the baby's bedside can help siblings better focus on the baby. Some distractions are removable whereas others are not, such as some of the medical equipment in or around the baby's bed. Siblings can be informed that they will see medical equipment, but it can be beneficial to remove or put away any unneeded equipment or supplies. Also, if the baby has a large number of toys around the bed, young siblings may want to play with them rather than interact with the baby. In this case, a few toys might be left out and the rest put out of sight during the visit. Many siblings will look for any special toys they have picked out for the baby, so these should be displayed at the bedside.

Tip for Families

Toddler and preschool siblings can be easily distracted by a large number of toys in or near the baby's bed.

HELPFUL INFORMATION FOR THE HEALTH CARE TEAM

An awareness of certain issues before sibling visits can help the baby's health care team relate to and interact with siblings. Some of these issues are the number and ages of siblings in the family, as well as any diagnoses of development delays or learning differences. This knowledge provides caregivers with a better understanding of how siblings fit into their family unit, as well as how they cope and comprehend information.

Aspects of Siblings' Medical History

Bedside caregivers should also be aware of siblings' history of health care experiences. Some examples might be

- Frightening health care experiences or problems with regular or well-child physician or dentist visits

- Recent hospitalizations or emergency center visits for themselves, close family members, or friends

- Ongoing medical conditions such as cancer, diabetes, asthma, or chronic allergies

Some siblings with health-related experiences may be anxious about visiting the baby in a health care setting and need frequent reassurance about the safety of the baby and themselves in this environment. Other siblings with some of these experiences, however, may feel comfortable in the health care environment and in seeking information from members of the baby's health care team.

Siblings' Questions and Concerns

A prior knowledge of the issues recently discussed by the family can also help caregivers address siblings' questions or concerns about the baby and the NICU. In addition, caregivers should be aware of parents' comfort level about sharing information with siblings and take into consideration the family's cultural beliefs. Siblings' questions may include

- *"Is the baby in pain?"*—When siblings go to the doctor, they sometimes undergo painful procedures such as injections. They should be reassured that the baby's health care team is working hard to make sure the baby is not in pain.

- *"When the machine makes that sound, does it mean that the baby is going to die?"*—Often, the only reference siblings have of the hospital and especially critical care areas is what they have seen on television. When an alarm goes off in a medical show, something bad has usually happened or is about to happen. Siblings may need reassurance that the NICU is not like what they have seen on television and that sounds from medical equipment can mean different things.

- *"How can I help with the baby?"*—During the mother's pregnancy, families often discuss ways that siblings can help care for the baby. Siblings may be concerned that they will no longer be able to help now that the baby is in the NICU. The ways in which siblings can help care for the baby are highly dependent on the baby's gestational age, diagnosis, and condition. Even babies in a very critical condition can usually tolerate a sibling gently holding their hand or foot or kissing them on the forehead. Siblings can also make a special name sign or other artwork as well as choose a special balloon for the baby's bedside. As babies are able to tolerate more stimulation, siblings are able to provide more care such as choosing clothes or toys for the baby, helping hospital caregivers gather supplies the baby will need, talking or reading to the baby, holding the baby, or playing with the baby.

Families' Concerns

Families may be concerned about how siblings will react to the hospital environment or to the baby in the NICU. Research studies by Ballard et al. (1984), Oehler and Vileisis (1990), and Schwab et al. (1983) have found that siblings who were able to visit the baby in the NICU viewed it as a positive experience and often had better coping skills than siblings who were not allowed to visit. They also reported that after their first visit, siblings often said they would like to visit again. Another concern of parents may be their difference of opinion with others about sibling visitation issues. Parents may need assistance and support responding to family members or friends who disagree with their decisions about allowing siblings to visit and interact with the baby in the NICU.

Families may also be concerned about infection risks for the baby. Kowba and Schwirian (1985), Solheim and Spellacy (1988), Umphenour (1980), and Wranesh (1982) reported no increase in bacterial infections following sibling visitation of healthy newborns in a maternity setting when sibling health-screening and hand-washing policies were followed. Ballard et al. (1984), Hamrick and Reilly (1992), and Schwab et al. (1983) reported no increase in nosocomial infections in infants following sibling visitations in the NICU when visiting siblings were screened for communicable diseases and followed current unit infection control policies. Siblings and other family members should not visit the baby when they are sick, as this could put their baby's health or the health of babies nearby at risk.

SIBLING PREPARATION

Siblings should be prepared before they visit the NICU to help reduce misunderstandings and misconceptions. When to prepare siblings for visits often depends on siblings' developmental level. Because toddler and preschool siblings can have difficulty understanding the concept of time, they should be prepared the day of their visit. School-age, preteen, and adolescent siblings should be prepared in advance to allow them time to process the information they have been given and to ask questions. It is also important to prepare siblings in consultation with their family, which allows parents to retain their parental role and to have an active part in the process. To further assist with the preparation process, families might be offered individual consultations; information by way of fact sheets, pamphlets, books, coloring books, and the hospital's web site; and videos and DVDs. The baby's health care team can then reinforce this preparation and address any additional questions and concerns siblings may have when they come to visit the baby.

Tip for Families

The best time to prepare siblings for visiting the baby often depends on the siblings' developmental level.

Approaches for Preparation

One way to prepare siblings is by using the sensory approach, that is, explaining in developmentally appropriate language what they will see, hear, smell, and possibly feel while they are in the hospital. Following are some of the sights, sounds, smells, and textures that siblings might need to be prepared for.

Sights

- Appearance of the baby compared to that of babies they have seen in the past
- Members of the health care team they might meet and the types of clothes they will be wearing, such as various-colored scrubs, white coats, or gowns over their clothes
- Equipment around the baby's bed space or attached to the baby
- Type of bed the baby is in
- Size of the NICU and approximate number of babies in the NICU or around the baby's bed

Four-year-old Theo has experienced several hospitalizations and emergency center visits for asthma. When he saw a picture of his baby brother in the NICU with a nasal cannula, he became excited and said, "The baby is just like me at the hospital."

Sounds

- Beeps and other sounds from equipment near the baby's and other babies' bedsides
- Hiss of air and oxygen through tubing
- Interactions of other families with their babies
- Emotional reactions of other families
- Hospital caregivers talking to one another and to other families
- Babies crying and cooing

Smells

- Different types of medication
- Baby's wet or dirty diapers
- Various cleaning supplies
- Baby lotion and shampoo

Textures

- Type of hand-washing soap

- Baby's skin

- Blanket on baby's bed

- Items in baby's bed used for positioning or to help prevent skin breakdown

Another way to prepare siblings is by using a step-by-step or time-line approach, in which events are explained to siblings in a sequential fashion. Combining the sensory approach and the step-by-step or time-line approach offers siblings the benefits of both. Another approach, which can also be used with the others, is the role-model approach, in which the baby's family or caregivers act as a positive role model for siblings in such areas as interacting with the baby, hand washing, or reacting to the hospital environment.

Preparation for Events Before Bedside Visits

Siblings need to be prepared not only for what they may experience at the baby's bedside but also for events that take place before they see the baby. One of these is hand washing. The big scrub sinks in some NICUs can be overwhelming for young siblings, especially if they are hard to reach and step stools are not provided. They may need explanations about the importance of hand washing and infection control regarding the baby. Siblings also need to be prepared for aspects of their health screening, such as having their temperature taken with a thermometer that might look different from the one used at home. For some siblings who have a history of frightening health care experiences, this can be upsetting. Siblings who have been told by their parents that if they misbehave the doctor will give them a shot may think that the unfamiliar thermometer will be used for an injection. Siblings may also need preparation for the brief wait while their family is questioned about their illness history or immunization record, as it can be difficult for siblings to wait when they are eager to visit the baby.

Rozdilsky (2005) discussed that siblings who are restricted from visiting because of problems shown in their health screening may

---

Tip for Families

If siblings are frightened about having their temperature taken, allowing them to role-play by taking a doll's temperature can be beneficial, as well as providing a thermometer that looks like the one they use at home.

need developmentally appropriate explanations about why they are un-able to visit. She suggested telling them that they will be able to visit at another time, reassuring them that they have not caused the visit to be postponed, and providing them with alternative ways to be involved with the baby.

Preparation for Interacting with the Baby

Most siblings have had no experience interacting with a baby in the NICU. They will need to be prepared to interact without overstimulating or hurt-ing the baby or disturbing any medical equipment such as intravenous (IV) lines, nasogastric (NG) tubes, or endotracheal (ET) tubes. Young siblings who may have been expecting a playmate may need assistance to help them understand that the baby is smaller and more fragile than they are and needs to be treated gently and tenderly. Opportunities can often be pro-vided for siblings to interact with the baby even when the baby is critically ill, such as placing a finger in the baby's hand or holding the baby's toes or feet. Siblings may also need assistance in learning the baby's cues. As the baby grows and develops and its cues change, siblings will need to continue to learn ways of interacting.

Preparation for Preschool and School-Age Siblings

Because visiting the baby in the NICU may be the first time that siblings have visited a family member in a hospital or an intensive care unit, they may need developmentally appropriate explanations regarding the type of be-havior expected in the hospital setting. These expectations are better re-ceived when stated in a positive rather than negative manner, such as

- "Please use your inside voice or whisper voice inside the hospital. Loud voices can disturb the babies who are trying to sleep."

- "It's important to be quiet inside the NICU. Many of the babies are try-ing to sleep. This is their bedroom while they are in the hospital."

- "It's important to stay near your baby's bed. The other babies may be sleeping and they need their rest."

- "Thank you for trying to be quiet."

- "Thank you for walking."

- "I appreciate your behavior."

It is also beneficial to reinforce siblings' positive behaviors and redirect neg-ative behaviors. Ways to redirect rambunctious siblings include asking them about events in their life such as school, sports, friends, or favorite television shows or providing crayons and paper to allow them to take a short break and draw a picture.

> ## Tip for Families
>
> This may the first time siblings have been in a hospital, and they may not know what type of behavior is expected.

Preparation for Preteen and Adolescent Siblings

Preteen and adolescent siblings mature at different rates, which can affect their preparation needs, so it is important to consider the individual sibling when providing information. They may still have misunderstandings and misconceptions but may hesitate to ask questions or voice concerns. They may nod yes or say yes even when they do not understand the questions being asked. Appearance can be very important to siblings of this age, and they do not want to appear stupid or ask stupid questions.

These siblings are often aware of how the baby's diagnosis and hospitalization are affecting their family. Therefore, they may not want to ask certain questions in front of their parents or discuss concerns if their emotions and opinions are different from their parents' and other family members'. Some may need opportunities to discuss issues with members of the baby's health care team away from their family, but prior permission should be received from their parents.

DURING VISITS

Siblings' attention span can vary according to their developmental level, temperament, and stress level. Families and the baby's health care team need to be aware of when siblings become restless, rambunctious, or lose interest and be able to intervene appropriately, such as redirecting siblings or ending the visit. The baby's cues should also be monitored during sibling visits to help reduce problems such as overstimulation. Siblings also need information about how the baby is responding to their visit and how to read the baby's cues.

Siblings should be permitted time to get to know the baby in their own way. Depending on their temperament and comfort level, some siblings may go to the baby's bedside immediately, whereas others may need time to warm up to the environment and situation. Anderberg (1988) reported that siblings should be allowed to become acquainted with the baby at their own pace before being asked to touch or kiss the baby or pose for pictures. She stated that these requests can disrupt bonding behaviors between siblings and healthy newborns during the sibling's first visit in the hospital setting. She also reported that siblings who had had experiences with loss or death showed fewer bonding behaviors than siblings who had not had these experiences.

Communicating with the Health Care Team

Brazy, Anderson, Becker, and Becker (2001) reported that primary or consistent nurses can help parents feel more comfortable in the NICU. Being able to see and interact with familiar and trusted members of the baby's health care team can also help make the NICU a more comfortable place for siblings when they visit. Consistent members of the health care team not only have an opportunity to learn about the baby's issues, but also about the family's and siblings' issues. They may become familiar with siblings and learn more about their concerns. They are also able to include siblings to a greater extent in the baby's hospitalization and discharge process. Young siblings may enjoy creating artwork for particular caregivers with whom they have developed a special relationship. Consistent or primary health caregivers can also help parents feel more comfortable about leaving the baby and spending time with siblings away from the hospital.

Utilizing Siblings As Translators

Some families may use a primary language other than English in their homes, and the adults may not speak English well or at all. They may have a history of utilizing their children to communicate with the English-speaking world. Free, Green, Bhavnani, and Newman (2003) and Green, Free, Bhavnani, and Newman (2005) interviewed preteens and adolescents from several nationalities and stated that there were benefits and disadvantages to having them interpret for family members. Their experiences with translating in the health care environment were for the most part brief and uncomplicated, but at times became more complex as a result of the sensitive nature of some issues and possible difficulties with vocabulary, accents, and nonverbal communication. Many of them had experienced at least one unfavorable encounter. Free et al. and Levine, Glajchen, and Cournos (2004) also reported that when children are placed in the role of interpreter on a regular basis, they can miss important developmental activities such as school and extracurricular activities.

Opinions differ on whether family relationships and roles can change when children take on the role of translator. Ngo-Metzger et al. (2003) stated that when siblings are used as translators, relationships have the potential to change within the family because its younger members can be placed in a position of decision making. Green et al. (2005)

reported that children's assistance with translating does not change or interfere with family roles.

Laws, Heckscher, Mayo, Li, and Wilson (2004) discussed that children who act as interpreters in the health care setting may not always be treated the same as other interpreters because they are children. Some of their questions and responses may be ignored or diminished because they are not considered as important as adult questions and responses. Their questions and responses, however, may often be originating from an adult family member. Free et al. (2003) reported that when a problem occurred during the translation process, health care professionals tended to believe that the fault was with the translation rather than that the adult was not agreeing with their information. They also reported that children who act as interpreters can feel ignored if health care professionals do not provide eye contact during communication, and recommended that communication be directed toward the child to help the child feel involved and included in the experience.

Tip for Families

Siblings can have difficulty when they are consistently utilized as translators in the NICU.

Sibling Safety Issues

Young siblings need to be supervised while they are in the hospital, both inside and outside the NICU. Some parents may leave siblings unsupervised outside of the NICU when they become restless during their visit at the baby's bedside, which can pose a significant safety risk for siblings. Hospital elevators, stairwells, and hallways can be tempting places for young siblings to explore and easily become lost. Also, some families may become so comfortable in the hospital setting that they can forget they are in a public building with many exits that children can slip out. Also, parents have no control over who comes and goes in the hospital.

Another safety issue for siblings in the hospital can be some of the furnishings. For example, young siblings may need to stand on a chair to reach the sink to wash their hands or to reach the baby's bed level to see and touch the baby. Some chairs in the hospital swivel or have wheels, making them especially dangerous for wiggly young siblings to kneel or stand on. If these chairs are the only option, it is important that an adult who is able to pay close attention stands next to the sibling. This can be difficult for some family members because when the baby appears to need something, their attention can easily be drawn away from the sibling.

Being Asked to Leave the NICU

Occasionally during visits, siblings may be asked to leave the baby's bedside for a while because of a procedure that the sibling should not witness or an emergency elsewhere in the NICU. Siblings can misunderstand or misinterpret the reason they had to leave and may believe that they somehow caused the event or that caregivers are not being truthful with them. Explaining to siblings why they were asked to leave, what will happen to the baby while they are gone, and when they should be able to return is beneficial. If siblings appear anxious, they should be reassured periodically that they have not been forgotten. When siblings return, it is important to follow up with a quick synopsis of what happened to the baby while they were gone.

Tip for Families

If siblings are asked to leave the NICU because of a procedure or an emergency, they need honest, developmentally appropriate explanations to help prevent misunderstandings.

Siblings may also be asked to leave the NICU for a code situation, which can be a frightening and confusing experience. Some siblings watch a variety of medical shows on television, which has the potential to affect how they perceive this experience. Gordon, Williamson, and Lawler (1998) reviewed CPR survival rates on several British television shows that appeared to be close to the rates at a number of British hospitals. Diem, Lantos, and Tulsky (1996), however, looked at the CPR survival rates on several popular television medical shows in the United States and reported that the rates were significantly higher than those reported in the literature. They also discussed that on television the outcome following CPR was either survival or death and that disabilities were rarely shown. Baer (1996), in response to the Diem et al. (1996) study, reported that television shows are drama and that physicians need to provide more information to their patients about CPR.

Van den Bulck (2002) reported a significant relationship between adolescents watching a popular Flemish medical drama that showed CPR and overestimation of survival rates for CPR in a hospital setting. Also discussed was that adolescents may judge medical professionals' behaviors during CPR based on what they have observed on television. Van den Bulck and

Damiaans (2004) compared cardiac arrest rates in this same Flemish medical drama and found that the rates were close to reality. These medical programs, however, can send the message that cardiac or respiratory arrest do not have to mean automatic death and that medical intervention has the potential to save a person's life.

Siblings often have fewer life experiences than adults and may have a more difficult time separating the CPR they see on their favorite television medical drama from the CPR they observe in the NICU. When they observe a code situation happen to their baby or another baby, they need to be reassured that the baby's health care team is doing everything possible to help the baby.

Exposure to Other Families in the NICU

Siblings visiting the hospital are often exposed to families of other babies, in both the NICU and waiting room. They can observe family and cultural differences in the ways that different families cope with their NICU experience, including religious and cultural rituals related to the birth, hospitalization, or death of a baby. Siblings may often need assistance to understand these differences.

Due to the serious nature of patients' conditions in many critical care units, siblings may observe families experiencing grief on various occasions. Johnson (1997) reported that families may observe the NICU unit routines that occur in response to a critical event or death. She also reported that the families who are visiting their children often support and share information with each other that is not shared with the health care team. Siblings who have the potential to overhear some of the conversations of these families may develop further misconceptions and misunderstandings.

ENDING THE VISIT

Some siblings can have difficulty saying good-bye to the baby and leaving the NICU. Allowing them to end their visits when they are ready can make it easier for them, although this may not always be feasible. Siblings may need reassurance that the baby will continue to be well cared for and that they will be able to visit again. They may also have questions concerning when the baby will be able to come home. Possible ways to support siblings when it is time for the visit to end are taking a picture of siblings and the baby together for siblings to keep; scheduling siblings' next visit; or giving siblings homework, such as bringing something special for the baby the next time they visit. Homework items might be a picture of themselves, artwork, a special toy, a small stuffed animal, a soft blanket, socks, or a hat. These assignments give siblings a specific reason to leave the NICU as well as to return.

Providing follow-up after visits helps siblings process what they have experienced and provides opportunities for them to ask their final questions. It also gives the health care team a chance to clear up misconceptions and misinterpretations before siblings leave the NICU. When families are included in these conversations, members of the heath care team can serve as role models regarding the importance of discussing these issues with siblings. Sometimes siblings may not have much to say, and at other times they may be regular chatterboxes. Siblings may also be too overwhelmed from their visit, too apprehensive, or too embarrassed to show emotions in an unfamiliar environment in front of unfamiliar people. If they have been told to be on their best behavior if they want to visit the baby again, this can inhibit their responses as well.

Tip for Families

Provide follow-up for NICU visits even after the family has left the hospital. Issues that families might discuss with siblings are their favorite part of the visit, what happened during their visit, whether they want to visit again, and how they can continue to be involved.

MAKING SIBLING VISITS
SUCCESSFUL AND MEMORABLE

There are several ways to help make sibling visits to the NICU memorable and to make siblings feel welcome at the baby's bedside. One is to encourage the family to bring a few family photographs to hang near the baby's bedside, which can help identify the baby as a member of the family and also help siblings find the baby's bed space. Families should be encouraged to bring photographs that can be easily replaced in case they are accidentally lost.

Also, taking pictures during sibling visits on a regular basis can help create a time line of the baby's hospitalization for siblings. It can help them remember how tiny or sick the baby used to be and how far the baby has come since admission. It also provides visual reminders that can make it easier for siblings to talk about their visits with family and friends. Another way to identify the baby as a member of the family is to take periodic family photographs that include the baby with the entire family or various family groupings. Some siblings may enjoy taking pictures of the baby with their own camera during visits, but may need to be reminded to only take pictures of their baby and not other babies in the NICU.

Artwork

Young siblings often enjoy sharing their artwork with important people in their life, which can include the baby and possibly members of the health care team. Displaying their artwork or schoolwork near the baby's bed can also help them find their baby's bed space when they visit. Some siblings create a large amount of artwork, which may need to be rotated. Some sibling artwork can be overstimulating for the baby. If this is an issue, artwork should be displayed so that it is out of the baby's eyesight but still visible to the sibling.

Certificates

A special visitation certificate that siblings can share with friends and classmates can often help them feel special and recognized. Certificates could be created on and printed from a computer or made on preprinted certificate paper. These certificates could also serve as an inexpensive marketing device for the hospital or NICU. Montgomery et al. (1997) suggested adding to the certificate the baby's handprints or footprints or both and a photograph of the sibling and baby taken during the visit. They also mentioned that siblings can use the certificates as a way to share information with others. Some siblings may want to add their own handprints to the certificate to be able to compare them in size to the baby's. If handprints or footprints are used, it is important to recognize the baby's overstimulation cues when taking the baby's prints, especially if they are taken on a regular basis.

Family Time at the Baby's Bedside

The hospitalization of a baby can limit the amount of time a family is able to spend together as a family unit. Activities that families can share in together at the baby's bedside can help siblings integrate the baby into their family. Some activities that have the potential to promote family interaction with the baby include playing with the baby, reading stories, and praying together, or taking care of the baby together. Families should consider siblings' developmental level as well as the amount of stimulation the baby can tolerate.

Sibling Activities in the NICU

There are times during visits when siblings will need to wait, such as to have their health screen completed, while their parents talk with other families, while the baby sleeps, or after they have visited the baby. Some siblings will have difficulty waiting quietly and can often benefit from developmentally appropriate toys and activities either from home or provided by the hospital. Suggestions for quiet hospital toys or activities might be

- Games that do not require materials, such as I Spy and The Quiet Game

- Pencil and paper games such as Tic-Tac-Toe or Hangman and activity books

- Books and children's magazines

- Art materials such as crayons, markers, or stickers

- Card games and travel games

- Cars, trucks, dolls, Legos, and small figurines

- Electronic games with mute buttons

- CD or MP3 player with headphones

Tip for Families

It can often be beneficial to periodically rotate toys and activities to maintain siblings' interest and reduce boredom, especially if the baby is hospitalized for a long period.

Normalizing the Baby's Environment

Siblings can often have a role in normalizing the baby's environment, which can benefit the baby's development as well as support the baby's transition home. Items that can assist with siblings' involvement include

- Mylar balloons to decorate the baby's bedside (Some siblings may want to pick out a special balloon for themselves as well. Mylar balloons are suggested because the American Academy of Pediatrics and U.S. Consumer Product Safety Commission recommended that latex balloons not be used around children younger than age 8. Many children's hospitals have banned latex balloons in part because of these recommendations.)

- Small, soft stuffed animals to assist with the baby's positioning

- Soft blankets to help keep the baby warm while being held

- Hats, booties, and other clothes for the baby to wear

- Toys for the baby to play with

- Books, lullaby tapes, or CDs

Before picking out any gifts, check to make sure these items are allowed in the NICU.

Siblings can also join in creating a family audiotape that can expose the baby to some of the voices of various family members when they are away. To create this tape, the family can read to the baby, send the baby special messages, or just let the tape run during family routines such as mealtime or during different aspects of the sibling's bedtime routine. This can also be a wonderful way for families to introduce some of the home environment and routines to the baby while the baby is still in the hospital.

Tip for Families

Some babies in the NICU can be overstimulated by a having a story read or tape played over and over. If the baby is able to tolerate the stimulation for a short period, the time can be gradually increased.

Holidays

Families with children tend to enjoy celebrating holidays that are important in their culture and faith. To create memorable visits around holiday times, families may want to include the baby in various aspects of their family holiday celebrations. One suggestion might be to decorate the baby's bed or bed space for the holidays. Each NICU has its own guidelines about the types and number of decorations permitted, which should be communicated to families. Families should be reminded not to bring items that are irreplaceable or that they would not want to be lost or broken. Some items for decorating the baby's bed and bed space might be

- Pictures of siblings and of the entire family participating in the holiday celebration or preparing for the holiday

- Plastic window clings in holiday or seasonal designs

- Small items from the holiday celebration, such as an artificial Christmas tree, stuffed Menorah, stuffed Easter bunny or Easter basket, or the baby's Halloween costume

- Blankets with holiday designs to place on the baby's bed

These suggestions may need to be modified depending on the baby's fragility or issues with skin integrity, temperature control, or positioning.

CONCLUSION

Sibling visitations have the potential to provide a variety of positive experiences for siblings and their families. They can also provide information to the health care team that would be difficult to get in any other way. Many siblings have no or limited experiences in critical care units, so preparation is important prior to visits to the NICU, especially the first visit. Follow-up support is also beneficial to help clear up any misconceptions or misunderstandings siblings may have. Visits to the NICU can help siblings not only become acquainted with the baby but also begin a positive lifelong relationship with their new brother or sister.

7

Coping with the Birth and Hospitalization of the Baby

How to Help Siblings

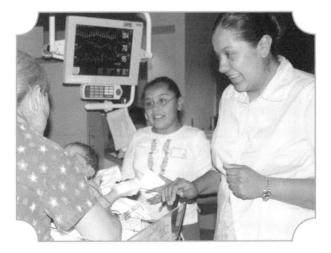

A new baby hospitalized in the NICU can be a life-altering experience for every member of the family, including siblings, but it can also be a growing and learning experience. There are opportunities to participate in new events, meet new people, and face new challenges. It is often beneficial when parents have awareness of siblings' coping skills and are able to share this information with others.

FACTORS AFFECTING HOW SIBLINGS COPE

The number of children in the family and where siblings are in the sibling group can affect coping. Siblings may be able to assist and support one another as they cope with the baby's birth and hospitalization as well as other changes that may occur during this time. This support system can be especially beneficial during difficult times when parents are unable to provide assistance and support for reasons such as physical distance, emotional distress, or grief. Siblings can also utilize other siblings as role models on how to appropriately respond to different aspects of the baby's hospitalization. In addition, siblings can help reduce one another's feelings of isolation in that they are going through the same experience together.

Most siblings have had routine health care, and some have had emergency center visits, hospitalizations, or visits with loved ones in the hospital. These experiences can influence how they perceive and cope with aspects of the baby's birth, such as visiting their mother and the baby in the hospital.

Rico had a difficult time receiving several painful injections during his 2-year well-child checkup. One month later, his parents showed him a picture of the baby in preparation for his first visit to the NICU. He began to scream, "No shots; no shots!" The nurse in the photograph was wearing scrubs that were the same color as those of the nurse who had given him the injections.

Lily, who is 3, was hospitalized for a brief time 4 months before her baby sister was born. The most difficult part of Lily's hospital experience was getting an intravenous (IV) line. When she peeked into the NICU to see her baby sister for the first time, she found a nurse starting an IV on a baby nearby. Believing that she would be next, Lily refused to go into the NICU and wanted to leave the hospital immediately. Lily's mother assured her that big sisters do not get IVs in the NICU. She also arranged for Lily to have lunch with the baby's consistent bedside caregivers in the hospital cafeteria to help her feel secure and comfortable enough to visit the baby again.

George had a tonsillectomy 2 years ago as a 2-year-old. His mother, a single parent, was unable to be with him when he woke up after the surgery because she had no one to stay with her 6-month-old son. George refused to visit his new baby sister in the hospital and began to cling to his mother, seldom letting her out of his sight. He equated the hospital experience with being separated from his mother and wanted to make sure he was not separated from her again.

Five-year-old Emma recently experienced the death of a grandparent and an elderly neighbor in the hospital. She has concerns that her new baby brother who is hospitalized in the NICU will die, too, even though her mother has told her on several occasions that he should be home in a few weeks. Emma informed her kindergarten teacher that "hospitals are where you go to die."

Many siblings have developed coping skills for difficult situations well before the baby's hospitalization, but these skills may not be appropriate for their current situation. They can need assistance and support to adapt their coping skills or to learn new ones, especially if the baby's hospitalization is long or the baby develops a chronic condition. Because children often do better with concrete, rather than abstract, suggestions and assistance, Espeland (1998) recommended providing them with clear and specific suggestions on coping issues, as well as taking cultural matters into consideration.

It is also helpful to observe how other members of the family are coping. Children tend to take cues from important adults in their life and will often imitate other family members' coping skills. If family members are coping in a positive, confident, and assured manner, siblings are likely to do the same. It can be challenging for some parents when siblings' coping needs are different from their own. It can also be difficult for parents when siblings' coping needs begin to change, such as when the baby's hospitalization progresses, the baby's medical status changes, the sibling matures, or the level of family stress changes. Families may need more assistance during these times.

Eight-year-old Cheyenne was very excited when her baby sister was born. She visited her in the NICU with their parents several times per week and actively participated in her care. As her sister's hospitalization progressed from weeks to months, Cheyenne's excitement began to decrease, and she began to visit her sister less frequently in order to spend time with her friends. Her mother had great difficulty with this change. She felt that it was very important for the family to spend time together. The neonatal child life specialist discussed with

her the importance of peer relationships for 8-year-old girls as well as the importance of maintaining Cheyenne's routines during the baby's extended hospitalization. Cheyenne continued to visit her sister several times per month with her parents, but she was also able to participate in baseball games, ballet lessons, birthday parties, slumber parties, and trips to the mall with friends.

Terry and Hailey, who are 9 and 12, visited their baby brother in the NICU on a regular basis with their parents. Several weeks after the baby's birth, their father decided that a sick baby in the NICU was more than he could handle and left the family. The girls' mother was required to work more hours, and the girls were required to take on more responsibilities at home. Terry and Hailey began to resent these changes and wanted life to go back to the way it was. From their perspective, this was their brother's fault because he was the reason their father left.

CELEBRATION ACTIVITIES

There are a variety of activities that can help siblings cope with the baby's hospitalization, as well as help them celebrate the baby and their change in status to a new big brother or sister. Many of these activities facilitate family interaction and can be adapted to meet siblings' developmental needs and coping concerns.

Celebrating Siblings' Change in Status

As exciting as the addition of a new baby can be for most families, it can also be difficult at times due to some of the changes it can bring. One example for parents might be additional responsibilities along with extra time and energy needed to care for a new baby. An example for siblings can be their change in status, such as moving from being the only child to the oldest, or from being the youngest child to the middle sibling. Just as parents enjoy celebrating their parenthood through baby showers or passing out cigars, siblings can enjoy celebrating their change in status as well. They may want to share special big brother or sister cupcakes, cookies, or candy with their friends or classmates. Young siblings may want to wear big brother or sister T-shirts or buttons to visit their mother or the baby in the hospital as well as to preschool or center-based child care. Some siblings may even want to help create these. Other suggestions might be planting a big brother or sister tree they can watch grow, creating a big brother or sister certificate, or receiving an increase in allowance or additional privileges such as getting to stay up a little later.

Including Siblings in Sharing the News

After their baby is born, many parents want to share the exciting news, but they can be too stressed or preoccupied to do so when the new baby has been admitted to the NICU and his or her prognosis is uncertain. There are several ways to include siblings in sharing the news about the baby with others. Some siblings may want to be involved with the family's birth announcements, such as helping to pick them out, having their names included, or sending some to their friends and other special individuals. Other siblings may want to create their own announcements with crayons or markers or on the computer.

Leaving updates about the baby's progress on the family's answering machine, as discussed in Chapter 4, is another way for siblings to help share information. Some families may prefer creating a family web page that includes not only information about the baby, but also information about other family members. Siblings may be interested in helping with the web page, choosing information about themselves to include, or updating the baby's progress and other information as needed. Families that prefer having more control over who can access the information may be more comfortable using mass e-mailings, also discussed in Chapter 4. Many siblings have excellent computer skills and may volunteer to help create and send these mailings.

Photo Book

Siblings can enjoy having a variety of photographs of the baby to share with family, friends, and others in their community. Photo albums can help them keep track of these photographs and prevent them from becoming lost or damaged. Baby photo albums may hold up better under the wear and tear they will receive from very young siblings. Because babies tend to grow and change quickly, updated photographs should be added periodically. Siblings may also want to include photographs of their visits to the NICU where they interacted with the baby so that they can see how their role has changed over time. Pictures of the baby that siblings take with their own camera may give families and the baby's health care team some insight into the siblings' perception of this experience.

Book of Firsts

Each baby grows and develops at its own pace, but some babies in the NICU, especially those with long hospital stays, can have developmental delays. Many commercial baby books or calendars may, therefore, not apply to this population. A book of firsts is a way to create a unique baby book and record information about the baby for siblings and families. Types of information that might be included are

- First time different family members, including siblings, visited or held the baby

- Baby's first smile, bath, and haircut

- Baby's first time in a big bed and first time wearing clothes

- Baby's first time breast feeding or bottle feeding

- First holidays with the baby

The book of firsts concept can also be adapted for sibling issues. From the siblings' perspective, the baby's birth and hospitalization may not be the most important event occurring in their life or in their family during this time. Siblings' developmental issues continue even while the baby is in the hospital, and for some siblings there may be times when their issues take a higher priority than the baby's. However, there is often a potential in families for siblings' important events to be overshadowed by the baby's issues. For these reasons, it can be beneficial for some siblings to have their "firsts" or their important issues recorded or documented as well as the baby's. Some examples of firsts that may be significant to siblings are

- First time riding a bike, with or without training wheels

- First lost tooth

- First day of school

- First slumber party

- First day at camp

- First visit with the baby in the hospital

Other issues may include participation in school and extracurricular activities.

Time Capsule

A time capsule can be an enjoyable intergenerational project that families can put together to mark this special time in the history of their family. They may also enjoy adding items that mark accomplishments and interests of individual family members, including siblings. They may want to decide on a specific time for the capsule to be opened, or just bury it in the backyard or hide it in the attic for someone to find in the distant future. Adaptations might be creating a baby time capsule or a big brother or big sister time capsule.

Show and Tell at School

An important part of the school day for some children is show and tell, when they are able to share important aspects of their life with their friends and classmates. Some siblings may decide to share part of their family's NICU experience. Items they may want to share can include a picture of the baby and sibling together, as well as a baby diaper or pacifier. Various members of the baby's health care team may be able to provide other suggestions and assistance to help siblings with this project. After the baby is discharged and medically judged healthy enough, some siblings may be interested in taking the baby him- or herself to school for show and tell.

Sharing Relatives' Experiences as Children

Many siblings enjoy hearing about different family members' experiences as a baby or as a big brother or sister. This type of sharing can also be a way to promote interaction between siblings and different family members. Aunts, uncles, and grandparents can often have great stories about Mom or Dad as a baby or as a new big brother or sister. Siblings may also want to hear about and see videos that show how excited their parents were when they first learned they were pregnant with them, heard their heart beat, saw them for the first time, and other special aspects of their babyhood. Pictures and videos may help siblings understand that once upon a time they were very small and needed a great amount of time and attention from their parents, just as the baby does now.

Creating a Family Tree

After the birth of the baby, especially a baby admitted to the NICU, families can receive support from a number of different family members. Siblings may be unsure of who all these people are and how they are related to them. Drawing a family tree can help give siblings a visual idea of how everyone fits together and provides a visual reminder for them to refer back to as needed. Young siblings may benefit from the addition of family photographs to the family tree so that they can use it independently and will not have to rely on someone to help them read the names. Grandparents can be especially helpful with this activity because they usually know more relatives. Younger siblings may want to draw various pictures of their family, which may or may not include the baby.

Keeping a Journal

Older siblings can benefit from having a journal or diary in which to record their feelings about the baby and other matters. Writing about their feelings and other aspects of the baby's birth and hospitalization can help siblings cope. It also provides a place for them to list their questions and concerns about the baby's condition, diagnosis, or prognosis. Siblings should be allowed to choose their own journal and writing tools, such as pens, pencils, or markers. Some siblings may want to decorate their journal with stickers and stamps. As tempting as it might be, parents and other caregivers should respect siblings' privacy and not read their diary or journal without first obtaining permission. Some siblings may also want to write a story about their experiences as a big brother or sister of a baby hospitalized in the NICU.

Computer-savvy siblings may utilize the computer either off-line or online, for example, as a private or public blog, or possibly in a chat room as a way to express how they feel about the new baby. Parents may be too busy or stressed to closely monitor their children's computer use during this time and may need to be reminded that any information written on-line can be picked up by others (see Resources at the end of the book). Personal information discussed on-line, such as children being home alone on a regular basis while their parents are in a hospital visiting their baby, could place siblings' safety at risk.

CONCLUSION

The addition of a baby who is hospitalized in the NICU is often a new experience for many siblings. Some of their current coping skills may be effective to deal with this new experience, and some skills may need to be adapted. Siblings may need to learn additional skills as well. Parents are often used as role models by siblings as they cope with this and other potentially difficult situations, so it can be effective to support parental coping as well. It can also be effective to talk to parents about including siblings in family celebrations to acknowledge the addition of the baby to the family and to offer suggestions of celebrations that are child friendly.

8

Sibling Support Groups

Why They Are Important

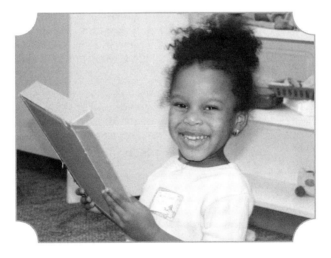

Sibling support groups provide opportunities for siblings in stressful situations to interact and connect with other siblings who have experienced or are experiencing similar situations. Siblings of hospitalized babies may not know anyone whose baby brother or sister was hospitalized, was diagnosed with an ongoing medical condition, or who may have died. Their peer role models for the big brother or sister role are likely to be friends whose mothers had healthy, full-term babies. These siblings may believe that theirs is the only family that has gone through an experience such as this, and some may begin to feel that they are different from their friends.

Support groups are often available for children who have a sibling diagnosed with an ongoing medical condition or disability or who have experienced a death in their family. In a few instances, support groups are also available for siblings of babies who are hospitalized in the NICU. In times of cutbacks and limited budgets, however, institutions and organizations may often limit the number of support groups they provide. As a result, siblings of babies in the NICU may be placed in a support group with siblings of children diagnosed with an ongoing medical condition or disability. Their experiences can be similar to those of the other children, although some aspects may be unique to their situation. These can include the addition of a new family member or their mother having health problems and possibly being hospitalized. These siblings can often benefit from opportunities to interact with other siblings of babies in the NICU during the baby's hospitalization.

In support groups, siblings can share coping strategies and discuss their feelings, thoughts, and experiences in a safe environment, which can help minimize feelings of isolation and loneliness. In addition, support groups can provide siblings with information that can help alleviate misunderstandings, misconceptions, or feelings of guilt. They can also provide parents with information on siblings' coping issues and possibly assist them with helping their children cope.

FAMILY ISSUES

Because families can define themselves in a variety of ways, they may need to determine for themselves who the baby's siblings are rather than relying on an institution's definition. In some homes, there may be children other than the baby's biological or adopted siblings who can be affected by the baby's hospitalization, diagnosis, or death. Cousins, young aunts and uncles, and other children can be affected as well and may need assistance and support to cope with the situation. These children, too, can benefit from participating in a support group.

Reluctance of Families to Participate in Sibling Groups

For various reasons, some families may hesitate to involve their children in a sibling support group. Strohm (2005) discussed that parents may be concerned about exposing their children to negative emotions and experiences of other siblings in the group. Weaver (1996) reported that families may believe that their child has been coping well and that interacting with siblings in the group could change this. She also stated that siblings can appear to be coping well but may be reluctant to discuss some issues with their family, especially issues that they feel may upset family members. For siblings who keep their thoughts and feelings bottled up, a sibling support group can provide them with a forum in which they can express their emotions in a safe, comfortable environment and learn ways to effectively express their emotions in other environments as well.

Tip for Families

Siblings who appear to be coping well can still benefit from a sibling support group.

Families that believe in "taking care of their own" may consider participation in a support group unnecessary. Parents who feel they are the experts on their children's issues may also be unreceptive to outside support. Some families may be concerned that their children will be exposed to information not in line with the family's cultural or religious beliefs, whereas others may have a negative history with support groups. Families that have had negative experiences with the social services system may believe that participation in a support group could put them at risk of being placed back in this system. Also, families that associate support groups with the mentally ill may discourage family members from attending for appearance's sake.

Some families may be concerned about the cost of support groups because of additional financial responsibilities associated with the baby's birth and hospitalization. The family budget may be in survival mode, with little left for "luxury" items such as sibling support groups. In some locations, sibling support groups are available at little or no cost, but hidden costs such as transportation and parents possibly losing work time and wages to transport siblings may prevent families from utilizing these services. Families may need additional assistance with these issues. Families may also hesitate or refuse to utilize these services if they view them as a charity. These families should be reminded that they are being charged the same as other participants or, if applicable, that the program is free of charge to all participants. Some of these families may be more inclined to participate if they are informed about ways to make donations or assist the organization in the future, which may help make these services seem less like a charity.

Family Support Groups

Siblings and their families can also receive support and assistance as they learn and interact together in family support groups. Siblings may observe not only how their peers cope, but also how adult family members cope. Family support groups and activity groups are available in many national organizations, some of which hold annual conferences where siblings and their families can gather with others for face-to-face support opportunities, even if a group is not located near their home.

CHOOSING A SIBLING SUPPORT GROUP

When deciding on a sibling support group, siblings and families should look for a group with a format or focus that best fits siblings' personalities. Different groups can have different areas of focus, such as socialization, reassurance, support, coping, education, communication, or diversion. Sibling support groups tend to have several areas of focus. When assisting families in choosing a group, it is beneficial to consider siblings' age, developmental level, temperament, and coping styles. It is also important to recognize that a group setting may not be appropriate for all siblings and that siblings should have a voice in deciding whether to become involved in a group.

The number, gender, and age of children who compose the group should also be considered. Some siblings may feel inhibited if there are too many or too few group members. They can feel lost in a large group of children, whereas their opportunities to meet and interact with others may be limited in groups that are too small. The number of group participants can also have bearing on the quality of supervision. With some siblings, the male–female ratio of the group may need to be considered. At some developmental levels, children are more comfortable in groups comprised of members of their own gender. If they happen to be the only girl or boy, or one of only a few girls or boys, they may not feel as relaxed, comfortable, or safe discussing certain issues. Ages of other group participants is another factor to consider. Many siblings feel more comfortable in groups in which participants are close to their own age. Some sibling support groups may be designed for specific age groups due to factors such as available resources, staff training, or meeting the needs of the majority of siblings.

Some sibling support groups provide opportunities for other family members to periodically participate in the group or to gain information. For instance, a staff person may be available to assist families with questions and concerns about sibling issues or to provide families with written information on a variety of topics. Other options might include educational programs for parents or family events such as picnics or family fun days.

STAFFING AND PROGRAMMING ISSUES

Before recommending a sibling support group to families, it is important to inquire about the skills and experience of the staff. They should have good communication skills with both children and families who are experiencing prolonged stress. They should also have a strong knowledge and understanding of child and family development and how this development can be affected by stressful events, such as having a new baby who is hospitalized, having a sibling with an ongoing medical condition or disability, or having a death in the family. Staff should also be able to observe and safely monitor all of the children and other individuals during the entire group meeting.

It can be helpful for siblings and families when the support staff is consistent and sibling support groups are regularly scheduled. Having a familiar staff helps siblings build a trusting relationship with staff members and other group participants. Also, because family routines may be changing during this time, a regularly scheduled sibling support group can become a reliable part of siblings' new routine.

Sibling support groups should also have planned goals and objectives as well as information on how they will be met. Some groups may have a formal vision and mission statement as well. This information can help determine whether a support group will be beneficial to a particular sibling or family. It can also help to identify which areas the group leaders believe are important, such as education, coping, support, or communication, as well as how programming will take place. Reports on group outcomes and responses from former participants may also be helpful.

LOCATING SIBLING SUPPORT GROUPS

Sibling groups can be found in a variety of settings. Some may be provided by the NICU or hospital. Munch and Levick (2001) described a side-by-side sibling parent group in the NICU during which parents were provided with information and suggestions regarding ways to support siblings, and siblings were given a format that focused on daily-life issues as well as assistance with support and coping issues. Lobato and Koa (2002, 2005) reported on Sib-Link, a side-by-side support group for parents and siblings of children with ongoing medical conditions or developmental disabilities that takes place in a hospital outpatient clinic setting. They reported that siblings showed increased knowledge of their brother or sister's diagnosis as well as increased feelings of connectedness. Sibling support groups can also be found in Ronald McDonald Houses, hospices, outpatient clinics, early childhood intervention programs, and other locations. Table 2 provides additional information on national and international sibling support groups.

Some siblings may feel more comfortable utilizing on-line support groups. Tichon and Yellowlees (2003) looked at SibKids to evaluate the

Table 2.   National and international sibling support groups

Program	Population served	Program history	Programming
The Sibling Support Project http://www.thearc. org/siblingsupport	Siblings of children with special health, mental health, and developmental needs	Developed by Don Meyer; based in Seattle, Washington	Face-to-face support groups (Sibshops) offered throughout the United States and other countries; on-line groups: SibKids and SibNet
Siblings Australia Inc. http://www. siblingsaustralia. org.au	Siblings of children with special needs	Established by Kate Strohm in 1999; based in Adelaide, Australia	Face-to-face groups based on the Sib-shop model available throughout Australia; on-line groups: SibChat4Kids, Teen-SibChat, and SibChat
The Dougy Center http://www. dougy.org	Children who have experienced the death of a loved one	Founded by Beverly Chappell in 1982; based in Portland, Oregon	Face-to-face groups offered in the United States and other countries

ability of an on-line sibling support group to provide assistance. They reported that emotional support, informational support, and social companionship could, in fact, be provided on-line.

On-line groups offer a variety of benefits. They can be accessed from home, which eliminates the need for transportation, and are usually available 24 hours per day, 7 days per week, which allows siblings to participate as their schedule permits. Many school-age, preteen, and adolescent siblings enjoy using e-mail and instant messaging to communicate with their peers as well as using the Internet to research new information. These methods of communicating can be especially appealing to them, as children in these age groups sometimes have difficulty sharing their thoughts and feelings with others face-to-face. They may also feel more comfortable communicating on-line because they can communicate when they feel they are ready and may have a greater sense of anonymity. This anonymity can be a disadvantage, however, in that siblings can miss out on opportunities to physically meet and interact with other siblings.

There can be other disadvantages to on-line groups as well. Younger siblings may not make the connection that they are communicating with another person as they type and receive information. Their only computer experience may be with computer games. Also, some siblings may not have developed the language, spelling, or fine motor skills needed to type on a computer keyboard, which can be frustrating for them. The cost of equipment needed to participate in an on-line support group, such as a computer and on-line connection, can be prohibitive for some families. They may need to consider utilizing a computer at school or at a local public library.

On-line support group web sites should be carefully reviewed before they are recommended to siblings and families. Information that siblings receive from these sites should be reliable, so web sites should be checked periodically for accuracy as well as for safety. On-line safety issues for children and teens should be discussed with family members, especially those who are new to the Internet, whenever on-line sibling support groups are recommended to families. For example, siblings should be advised not to give out certain information about themselves or their family or to arrange meetings with anyone they have met on-line without their family's permission. Also, families that are busy with the new baby may not always be aware of siblings' on-line activities. For safety reasons, families should look for groups that have a moderator, administrator, or web master or have restricted access. Families may also need assistance with creative ways to educate their children about on-line safety issues.

ADDITIONAL SUPPORT AND ASSISTANCE

Support groups provide opportunities for siblings to interact and communicate with other children who have had similar experiences, but Meyer and Vadasy (1994) and Strohm (2005) advised that support groups should not be regarded as therapy. Some siblings may need additional support and assistance to cope with the baby's issues and with changes that may be occurring in their family. Parents may request assistance and advice regarding behaviors that can signal a need for additional support. The American Academy of Child and Adolescent Psychiatry (2005a, 2005b) and The Dougy Center (2003) reported that some of the following behaviors may indicate a need for professional assistance:

- Persistent changes in eating and sleeping habits
- Persistent significant changes in school performance or refusal to go to school
- Persistent changes in behavior or activities, or isolation
- Persistent changes in interactions with others
- Changes in health, such as increased illnesses
- Decreased self-esteem
- Drug or alcohol abuse or both
- Sexual promiscuity
- Preoccupation with death or thoughts of suicide

Families may also request help in locating additional assistance or to receive a referral for services. Members of the baby's health care team who can make an official referral are physicians, nurse practitioners, and social workers. Some hospitals may have child psychiatrists and psychologists on staff who can also refer siblings or who may be able to provide the assistance themselves. Other individuals who may be able to help families and refer siblings for further assistance include the siblings' pediatrician, school counselors, or the family's minister or rabbi.

CONCLUSION

Siblings can receive numerous benefits from participating in sibling support groups. McMillan (2005) discussed the benefits her children received from participating in the Sibshop model of support groups. The Sibling Support Project recently surveyed some graduates of their support groups, Sibshops, and reported that more than 90% of those surveyed described the Sibshop experience as positive, and 94% would recommend it to others.

Although this format can benefit many siblings, it might not be the most effective way to provide every sibling with the support and assistance he or she needs. Families may hesitate to utilize a sibling support group for any number of reasons and may decide to look elsewhere, such as to their family, church, or friendship circles, for their support needs. If a sibling or family declines to participate in a sibling support group, the decision should be respected.

9

Multiple Babies in the NICU

Support for Big Brothers and Sisters

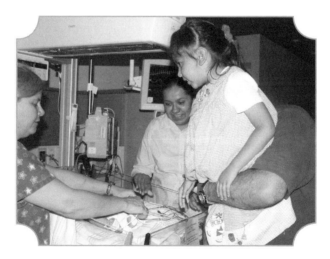

The number of multiple births has increased in recent decades. Reporting on the final birth data in the United States for 2003, Martin et al. (2005) stated that since 1980, the number of twins has increased by more than three quarters. They also reported that triplets and other higher-order births have increased more than 500% since 1980 but have remained stable since 1999. Blondel and Kaminski (2002); Martin et al.; and Russell, Petrini, Damus, Mattison, and Schwarz (2003) reported that increases in multiple births are the result of a growing use of fertility treatments as well as women having children later in life.

News of a multiple pregnancy can be both exciting and disconcerting for families. Just as with a single pregnancy, siblings should learn about the multiple pregnancy from their parents rather than from conversations they have overheard or from well-meaning family members or friends. Parents' conversations with siblings should be timed on the basis of siblings' developmental level, as well as on the health of the fetuses or the possibility of fetal reduction.

INCLUDING SIBLINGS DURING A MULTIPLE PREGNANCY

Siblings may enjoy helping their parents share the exciting news about the babies by telephoning, e-mailing, or text-messaging family and friends. Like other family members, siblings may want to talk to the babies and feel their movements. They may also enjoy discussing some of the differences between the babies, such as their gender, activity, position, and any possible health issues. An awareness of their differences can help siblings begin to view the babies as separate individuals.

Siblings can also benefit from being included in aspects of their mother's prenatal care. Listening to the babies' heartbeats or looking at the babies' ultrasounds can make the babies more real to young siblings. Occasionally during a multiple pregnancy, the number of babies may change, either because a baby who was hidden can now be seen or heard or because a baby has died. This information should be shared with siblings during the pregnancy, although in some cases it may not be known until the time of delivery.

Kamilah, age 4, was told that she would be a big sister to two babies in the middle of the summer. She was very excited and cuddled next to her mommy's tummy to tell the babies how anxious she was to see them. She also shared her favorite stories and songs with them. She enjoyed listening to their hearts beat and showed their ultrasound pictures to anyone willing to look. At some point during the pregnancy, one of the babies died, and Kamilah's mother gave birth to one healthy baby girl and one stillborn. Kamilah's father talked to her about the situation to help reduce her misconceptions and the likelihood that she would believe she caused the baby's death because of something she did, said, thought, wished, or prayed for.

Patrick's parents told him that triplets would be joining their family around Thanksgiving. His best friend had a new baby brother at home and informed 8-year-old Patrick that babies were disgusting—all they did was cry, poop, and drool. Patrick could not imagine what life would be like with three babies at home. He went with his parents early in the pregnancy to look at the ultrasound but otherwise was minimally involved in his mother's pregnancy. Over the summer during a routine ultrasound, another baby was located hidden behind one of the other babies. Patrick's parents were hesitant to tell him because of the way he had responded to the pregnancy with three babies. They waited until the babies' birth to inform him, but Patrick had a difficult time adjusting. Not only did he have to cope with the birth of the babies, but he also had to deal with an increase in the number as well.

Some siblings may enjoy and benefit from reading developmentally appropriate books about other siblings who have experienced multiple births in their family. The accuracy of these resources should be considered as well as how closely they match the siblings' and family's specific experiences. Some siblings and families may also enjoy telling or writing their own stories. Older siblings may want to utilize the computer, while younger siblings may prefer dictating a story to an adult and then illustrating it. These stories can provide insight into how siblings perceive the addition of multiple babies to their family but should not be read without first receiving the siblings' permission.

SIBLING COPING ISSUES

Because many people are interested in and curious about multiple births, especially higher-order births, multiple babies can attract a great amount of attention. Bryan (2003) and Campbell, van Teijlingen, and Yip (2004) discussed that siblings can often feel unnoticed, left out, and pushed aside when this occurs. Foley (1996b) mentioned that some siblings react by trying to seize extra attention for themselves. Haddon (2000) suggested that it can be helpful to tell people what a wonderful big brother or sister the babies have, as well as how wonderful and special all of the children in the family are. Some families may need suggestions and assistance with this issue.

Mr. and Mrs. Winter were enjoying a walk through their neighborhood with new triplets and their big sister, Shelby. On every block at least one person stopped to comment about the triplets in their stroller. Very few noticed that

Shelby was there. The neighbors' first comments were often, "Are they triplets? Aren't they cute." Shelby's parents learned to respond, "And this is their beautiful big sister," or "And this is our wonderful daughter."

Mr. Brown was shopping in the mall with his quadruplets and their 12-year-old sister, Chinara. The quadruplets in their stroller attracted a great deal of attention. Chinara began walking a distance away from her father and siblings and pretended she didn't know them.

While Ms. Claret was grocery shopping with her 4-month-old twins and their 3-year-old brother, Eli, they were periodically stopped by shoppers who commented on the twins and how cute they were. As this continued, Eli began to poke at the twins and finally tried to climb into their stroller on top of them. Ms. Claret responded to this behavior by creating a sign to hang on the stroller that read: "Yes, we are twins, and if you think we're cute, you should check out our big brother." She also asked Eli to help with the shopping by picking out certain items such as a box of cereal, a fruit, a vegetable, a package of cookies or crackers, ice cream, chips, and juice. This "big boy" job helped Eli feel special and provided a distraction when needed. It also introduced him to different types of foods he might not have tried otherwise.

Multiple births can also attract media attention. Because newspaper and television reporters will probably focus on the babies, parents should be reminded to include older siblings so that they do not feel left out or less important than the babies. Some siblings, though, may prefer not to be included because they do not want to appear different from their peers. Appearing in the newspaper or on television with their baby brothers and sisters may be uncomfortable or embarrassing for them.

SIBLING SUPPORT

There are a variety of ways to support sibling coping with the addition of multiple babies to the family, and most are identical to those used to help siblings cope with the addition of a single baby. Haddon (2000) discussed a few that are specific to siblings of multiple babies. These include not calling the babies "the twins," "the triplets," or "the quads" or dressing them in outfits that are alike, as this can cause siblings to feel isolated or excluded from the group.

Providing siblings with a variety of materials for pretend play can also be beneficial. Some examples are baby dolls in the same number and sex as the babies or a dollhouse with a doll for each family member, including the babies. If one or more of the babies needs medical equipment at home, the dolls can be adapted and the appropriate medical equipment added. Siblings' pretend play can also give families insight into how they perceive the new babies. If families have concerns about siblings' play, they may wish to

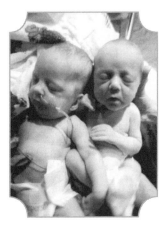

discuss them with the child life specialist, social worker, psychologist, psychiatrist, or the siblings' pediatrician.

Young siblings may enjoy wearing special shirts designed for big brothers and sisters of twins, triplets, or quadruplets. They can wear these shirts when they visit the babies or their mother in the hospital or when they are out with the babies. The shirts may also help draw attention to the sibling at a time when the babies are the center of attention. These shirts are usually available from local or Internet multiples clubs or from web sites. Some siblings may want to design and create their own shirts and possibly shirts for the babies.

Choosing special gifts for the babies or receiving surprises from the babies can be fun for siblings when they visit the babies in the NICU. To help siblings see the babies as individuals rather than as a group, siblings might choose a different gift for each baby and receive a different gift from each baby as well. If cost is an issue for families, gifts from the babies can be inexpensive, and gifts for the babies can be created by the siblings, such as a decorated framed picture of the sibling, a clay sculpture, a handmade or computer-made card, or a drawing or painting.

VISITING THE BABIES IN THE HOSPITAL

Locating multiple babies close together in the hospital can be helpful but sometimes challenging when the babies have different medical needs or a there is a high NICU census. In some cases, babies may need to be hospitalized in different areas of the hospital or possibly in different hospitals. This can make the situation even more difficult for parents when they are just beginning to learn to care for and interact with more than one baby at a time. When multiple babies are scattered throughout the NICU, siblings may be sent to see if one or more of the babies are awake or asleep while their parents are busy with the other babies. Parents can also become anxious when they hear repeated monitor alarms and may send siblings to check on the babies in other areas of the NICU. Locating the babies in proximity can eliminate the need to send siblings across the NICU. It can also make taking photographs of the babies together or with different family members much easier for families.

When the babies are located close together, families may need to be reminded to wash their hands and maintain other recommended infection control guidelines between handling each baby. When faced with several crying or upset babies, parents may forget about hand washing as they try to calm and soothe them all at once. Siblings who are excited to see the babies and move from baby to baby when they visit will also need gentle reminders to wash their hands before touching each baby. However, reminding them can often be difficult in a busy NICU. One effective method might be to create and attach a small sign to the babies' beds at siblings' eye level that serves as a reminder to wash their hands. Siblings might even enjoy helping to make these signs. An example might be a red octagonal sign with siblings' handprints and a slogan such as "STOP. Did you wash your hands?" Even siblings too young to read are often able to recognize the stop-sign shape and color and their handprint.

DEATH OF ONE OR MORE BABIES

The death of any baby is a devastating experience, but there are specific ways to help support families of multiple babies when one or more of them have died. Kollantai and Fleischer (1993) and Pector and Smith-Levitin (2002b) discussed that it can be very important to families that all of their multiple babies are recognized, even those who have died, no matter when they died. Calling two surviving triplets twins or surviving sextuplets quadruplets can send the message to families and siblings that those who died are not important or that they never existed.

Also, family members can have difficulty returning to the NICU where their babies died to visit the surviving babies, which can influence bonding and learning their care. Kollantai and Fleischer (1993) mentioned that some families can have further difficulty upon returning to the NICU when their surviving babies are located near a similar group of multiple babies who have all survived and when they observe families visiting the group. It can also be difficult for families to answer siblings' questions and concerns about death and dying while continuing to bond and interact with the surviving babies.

Another issue is photographs of the babies. When one or more of the babies is dying or has died, this is often the family's only opportunity for a photograph of the babies together or for a complete family photograph. For parents and siblings as well, these photographs can trigger important memories and become treasured additions to family photo albums. Kollantai and Fleischer (1993), Pector (2004), and Pector and Smith-Levitin (2002a) discussed how important these photographs can be for families. Pector and Smith-Levitin suggested that if photographing all of the babies together is not possible, a digital camera could be used to take separate photographs, which could then be arranged to create a group photograph of all of the babies. Pector (2004) suggested a family photograph could be taken with different family members holding different babies.

The ability to express their faith is important to many families during this time. Kollantai and Fleischer (1993) stated that families of multiple babies may want their babies baptized, christened, or blessed together. These rituals, which may include siblings, can provide families with cherished memories of the babies together. Kollantai and Fleischer also reported that families may wish to combine baptisms, christenings, or blessings for the babies who survived with memorial services for the babies who did not. If the surviving babies will be discharged soon, families may be able to schedule the combined ceremony at home. If one or more of the babies will be hospitalized for an extended time, families may prefer to schedule this service in the NICU or hospital chapel. Families may also need suggestions for ways to include siblings in these services.

SCHEDULES AND ROUTINES

Depending on the number of babies, some families may find caring for multiple babies easier when the babies are all on the same or similar schedules. The babies' schedules should be coordinated before discharge if possible, as this can be difficult to accomplish while making the transition to the home environment. Some families, especially those of lower-order multiple births, may prefer the babies to be on staggered schedules so that they can spend individual time with each baby. Siblings' schedules and routines may need to be considered and minimally changed, although this can be difficult with the addition of more than one baby to the family. A familiar, consistent caregiver may be able to assist with the continuation of siblings' routines and also provide siblings with assistance and support. This caregiver may also be able to help care for the babies so that parents can spend individual time with siblings as well. Foley (1996a) noted some ways to assist siblings of multiple babies to feel included, such as special activities and time together with their parents.

SUPPORT GROUPS FOR FAMILIES WITH MULTIPLE BABIES

Families can gain information and support on a variety of issues, including sibling issues, from their local twin or multiples club, where they can meet and interact with other families of multiple babies and learn how these families have handled certain issues. These groups can also be resources for hand-me-down sales or exchanges as well as for information about multiple babies. Families that may not want or have time to attend meetings may be interested in and more comfortable with interacting with families of multiple babies over the Internet. This may also fit better with their lifestyle or personalities. Several Internet groups from English-speaking countries such as the United States, Canada, the United Kingdom, and Australia are available. Before providing recommendations, it is important to critique these resources to see how well they fit a particular family's needs, as well as for accuracy of information and safety.

FOLLOWING DISCHARGE

The addition of multiple babies can be both time consuming and hectic for many families. Mariano and Hickey (1998) reported that it often takes more time and energy to care for multiple babies than many mothers anticipated during their pregnancy. As a result, they may not have planned for adequate assistance and support, which can be difficult to arrange while exhausted and caring for several babies as well as older siblings. The American Society for Reproductive Medicine (2003) reported that color coding babies' outfits and possessions can help families keep the babies straight. It may also help families stay organized and decrease the caregiving time required for each infant. If young siblings feel left out, they could be assigned a color as well. It can also be a challenge to get several babies and their siblings ready to leave the house and buckled into their car seats or stroller. Williams and Medalie (1994) reported that multiple strollers are helpful but because of their size may limit the places where families can go. Families can be further isolated if more than one adult is needed on an outing to help with the babies.

Family and Social Support

Because of their possibly different medical needs, multiple babies may be discharged from the hospital at different times. Parents can be stretched as they are adapting some of the babies to the home environment, visiting the rest of babies in the hospital, and supporting siblings as they adapt to changes in their environment caused by the babies' homecoming. Support from family and friends can be crucial to helping families cope. Extended family and family friends can help care for siblings and the babies at home so that parents can continue to visit the babies in the hospital. Assistance with caring for the babies at home can also allow parents to spend more time with older siblings as well as with each other.

Families can have differences in their ability and desire to seek or accept assistance. They may never have had to ask for assistance from others and may be reluctant to do so now. They may also have difficulty coordinating this assistance and eventually give up, believing it is easier to do things themselves. Other families may live a great distance from extended family members or may not have a good relationship with them. They can need help from the health care team to find long-term support and assistance in their local community as well as how to coordinate it.

Establishing Routines and Predictability

Once the babies are home, sibling and family routines often need to be adapted. This can be difficult for siblings who may feel overwhelmed by what they perceive as the invasion of the babies. Whenever possible, siblings should be given choices regarding how their routines or schedules will change. Extended family and family friends can also help with maintaining siblings' routines. Families might consider posting information about schedules and routines in a prominent place, such as the refrigerator or a kitchen cabinet, so it is visible to all caregivers. This information can be as detailed as parents wish to make it.

Designating a Baby-Free Space

After the babies are home, some siblings may feel that the babies have not only taken over their parents' time and attention, but that they and their paraphernalia are taking over the entire house as well. This impression can intensify if one or more of the babies have been diagnosed with special needs and require medical equipment or health care support at home. Creating a space designated for siblings that is free of babies and baby supplies can help reduce some of these feelings and give siblings a place to go when they need a break from the babies. As the babies grow and become mobile, this space may need to be reexamined to make sure it continues to be baby free.

Tip for Families

Several young toddlers leaning, pushing, pulling, or climbing on a baby gate at the same time can easily pull it out of the wall. If baby gates are used, they should be checked frequently.

Siblings' Assistance with Multiple Babies

Parents of multiple babies can have less time than they would like to interact with and care for each individual baby, and so may need assistance from siblings on a regular basis. Depending on their developmental level, siblings can help not only by playing and snuggling with the babies, but also by feeding and diapering them. When families ask siblings to keep an eye on several babies at the same time, they should consider the siblings' developmental level, the age of the babies, and the length of time they will be

Tip for Families

It is important that siblings are not made to feel they are gofers. Families should be aware of and avoid constantly interrupting sibling activities, homework, or play.

responsible for them. Families should also be encouraged to make siblings' assistance an option rather than a requirement.

CONCLUSION

The number of multiple births has greatly increased in the United States in recent years. The addition of more than one baby can be a hectic but wonderful event for many families. Siblings often benefit from opportunities to participate in many aspects of this experience. Families may need suggestions of different ways to include and assist siblings through various aspects of this experience.

10

Getting Ready for the Baby to Come Home

Including Big Brothers and Sisters

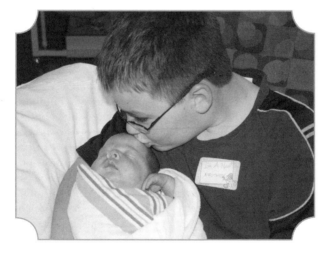

The baby's discharge from the hospital can be a happy but hectic time for families as they prepare to take their baby home. They often need to accomplish a great deal during this time, such as learning the baby's care and preparing for the baby at home. The American Academy of Pediatrics (1998); Ritchie (2002); and Verma, Sridhar, and Spitzer (2003) reported that when babies are discharged from the NICU, many may have ongoing medical needs. Parents may be required to become skilled at medical procedures they never imagined they would need to learn. With parents' attention focused on issues such as these, it can be especially important for the health care team to be cognizant of sibling issues during this time. Families may need suggestions for ways to include siblings in the discharge process as well as to prepare them for the baby's homecoming. Parents should be reminded to be aware of their own stress and exhaustion levels during this time, as their sleepless nights will significantly increase after the baby is home. Exhausted parents will be less likely to successfully cope with either the baby's or siblings' issues following discharge.

SIBLING SUPPORT

As parents prepare to take their baby home, their schedule can be more demanding than in the past, which means that they will have even less time to spend with siblings. Some siblings may be spending increased amounts of time with various caregivers, and a few may be spending more time in the NICU waiting room or at home alone. Talking with families about their child care decisions at this time can be beneficial.

In a few cases, caregivers may discover unsafe arrangements and be able to assist the family with this issue. In some families, an extended family member or family friend may move into the family's home for a short time to provide assistance and support before and after the baby comes home. For many families, this arrangement is an effective support system, but in others it can become a stressful situation. In a time of family mobility, siblings may have had limited contact with this individual with whom they are now expected to spend a large amount of time, and this can be distressing for them.

Some families may plan a special activity or vacation for siblings before the baby is scheduled to come home. It is helpful if the baby's health care team is aware of this plan so they can help coordinate it with the baby's discharge. If it appears that the baby will be discharged before the planned event, parents should be given enough time to reschedule. Many parents are more comfortable being away from the baby for this special activity or vacation if the baby's primary nurses can be scheduled to care for the baby.

SIBLING DEVELOPMENTAL ISSUES

It can be difficult for young siblings when the baby comes home and needs a great deal of their parents' time, attention, and energy. They need to be prepared for the baby's impending discharge and the changes that may occur after the baby is home, although they might find it hard to understand what this all means and how they will be affected, especially if the baby is their only sibling. Families may see some regressive behaviors similar to those the sibling displayed when the baby was born. It is often better to wait to begin new developmental tasks, such as weaning, potty training, moving to a "big kid" bed, or starting preschool until the baby has been home for a while. Young siblings can often benefit from continued opportunities to be included in the family's preparations for the baby's discharge. Ways to include them will often depend on factors such as the sibling's interests and abilities, the baby's care needs, and parents' comfort levels.

Paco, age 2, was excited that his new baby sister was almost ready to come home from the hospital. His father began to put the baby's crib together using some tools from his toolbox, and Paco had a great time helping with plastic tools from his own toolbox.

Three-year-old Mychau was watching her parents paint her baby sister's room in preparation for the baby's discharge from the NICU. She repeatedly asked to help, but because she had already stepped in the paint several times, her parents were hesitant. Instead, Mychau's mother provided her with lots of paper and watercolors. She gave Mychau clear instructions that the paints were to stay on the table and that after her paintings had dried, they would pick out a few to frame for the baby's room.

Gigi had been waiting a long time and was happy that her new baby brother was finally coming home from the hospital. During a visit with the baby in the NICU, she helped her mother prepare for the discharge by packing some of the baby's toys and clothes to take home.

Older siblings can also benefit from being included in the discharge planning. Some may be interested in participating with the baby's care; however, the baby's safety should always be the primary concern regarding sibling involvement. Older siblings can help parents, for instance, by distracting the baby while they provide medical care or by cuddling, playing with, or reading to the baby. Some siblings may also be interested in attending formal discharge planning meetings, which are usually scheduled and include members of the baby's health care team, or informal meetings at the baby's bedside. Depending on the length of these meetings, siblings may need to bring quiet activities, such as video games with mute buttons, word-search puzzles, or drawing paper, to keep them occupied if they become bored or

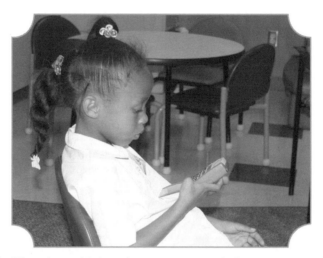

Figure 3: Siblings who attend discharge planning meetings may need to bring quiet activities to keep them occupied if they become bored or need a break.

need a break (see Figure 3). Support should be provided after these meetings to help dispel siblings' misconceptions and misunderstandings.

Ricky, age 7, was at his baby brother's bedside in the NICU with his parents while they were learning how to place a nasogastric tube. He brought his backpack, which contained his homework, several video games with mute buttons, and his MP3 player with headphones, to help keep him occupied. While he was there, several members of the health care team stopped by for an impromptu discharge planning meeting. Except for one member, the health care team ignored Ricky completely. This team member sat by Ricky and welcomed him as an important family member. She also encouraged him to ask questions and suggested ways he could be involved in the baby's discharge process.

Tanya and Jenna, ages 12 and 15, were excited about their baby sister coming home from the hospital in a few weeks. They had a slew of questions about how life would change at home and ways they could help care for their baby sister, and they asked their parents to attend the discharge planning meeting. They were greeted at the meeting as important members of their family and were encouraged to voice their questions and concerns. Follow-up was provided by their parents, the neonatal child life specialist, and the neonatal social worker, all of whom encouraged the girls to continue to share their questions and concerns as their family prepared for the baby to come home.

SIBLING COPING ISSUES

Families can have mixed feelings about taking their baby home. They may be happy about the baby coming home but can be sad about leaving relationships they made during the baby's hospitalization. Some of these relationships may have been with members of the health care team and other families they met in the hospital, who may have provided a great deal of support during the baby's hospitalization. Once the baby is discharged from the hospital, families will no longer see these people on a regular basis, and their relationship with them can change. Also, some families may believe that various members of the baby's health care team saved their baby's life, which can make saying goodbye or placing trust in another medical team difficult for them. Families can often benefit from being introduced to some of the health caregivers who will be available to provide care for their baby after discharge.

Siblings can also receive support from members of the baby's health care team as well as from siblings and other family members of babies hospitalized in the NICU. After the baby is discharged, siblings often lose these support systems. They may also lose support systems such as baby sitters or center-based child care teachers if one of the parents resigns from a job to stay at home with the baby or is at home for an extended time on Family Medical Leave. Families may decide that with a parent at home, siblings can be at home as well.

It can often be beneficial to discuss with siblings what they think life will be like after the baby comes home. Some may believe that family life will return to normal, meaning the way it was before the baby was born. Others may assume that their parents will be able to give them the same amount of time and attention as they have throughout the baby's hospitalization. Still others may wonder if their parents will have any time left over to spend with them. Most siblings will have difficulty predicting how much time and attention the baby will need from their parents and how life at home will change.

GETTING READY AT HOME

Some siblings will want to be very involved in the preparations for the baby at home, whereas others will not be interested at all. Siblings should be offered opportunities to participate and be allowed to decide how involved they want to be. Siblings can help prepare the baby's room and pick out special items such as toys, books, music, blankets, and clothes. Young children often do better when their choices are limited.

Tip for Families

When siblings are allowed to make choices, it is important to respect their decisions as often as possible. This helps them feel that they have been heard and that their thoughts and opinions matter.

Families may take a variety of photographs as they prepare for the baby at home. Including siblings in these photographs can be visual reminders of how important they were to the preparation process. Some siblings may want to assist or take their own photographs. What they choose to photograph can help families see what siblings viewed as significant in the process.

As families get ready for the baby at home, parents often sort through siblings' baby items for the baby to use. Siblings who may become upset about their baby things being given away without their consent should be allowed to choose a few items to keep for themselves. However, parents may need to pass down certain items, such as cribs, baby swings, playpens, strollers, high chairs, baby toys, or special holiday outfits. Some siblings who have chosen some of their baby items may want to keep them in a special place, whereas others may be satisfied with simply having been heard and given a choice in the matter.

The Sibling's Room

In some families, the sibling and baby will have separate rooms, and in others they will share a room. If the baby will have a separate room and it is being redecorated, siblings may feel left out and request to redecorate their room as well. Items for redecorating do not have to be expensive or elaborate. Some possibilities might be a set of sheets with their favorite characters, special pillows for their bed, a bedside lamp, a rug, or bookshelves. If siblings will be sharing a room with the baby, their space should be separate from the baby and the baby's possessions. Siblings may want to decorate this space in a way that identifies it as their own.

Planning a Homecoming Celebration

Families can celebrate the baby's homecoming in various ways, and siblings should be included in these activities whenever possible. An example might be using special banners or signs to welcome the baby home, which can be placed in front of the house or in the baby's room. Siblings may enjoy helping to create these signs as well as placing them around the house. Families may also plan special family get-togethers or special meals. Siblings may want to add some of their favorite foods to the menu, and older siblings may want to help cook the meal.

SUPPORTING THE BABY'S TRANSITION HOME

Families may need suggestions of ways to support the baby's transition from the hospital to the home environment, as well as ways to include siblings in the process. Differences between the environments may include visual, auditory, tactile, and olfactory stimulation, along with changes in temperature and daily routine. Families may want to bring a few of the baby's items from home to help with the transition process, such as bedding, which can have a different feel and smell from bedding at the hospital. Siblings can help choose special items such as blankets, toys, and clothes for the baby to use in the hospital so that the baby will be familiar with them following discharge.

Siblings may also enjoy helping their family make audiotapes for the baby to listen to when family members are not around. On these tapes, siblings can talk to the baby about the exciting things they anticipate doing with the baby after discharge or fun things they are currently doing, or they can read the baby special stories. Families could add to the tape during mealtime or bedtime routines, as more family members, including siblings, might be present.

THE BABY AND FAMILY ROUTINES

Parents should be encouraged to introduce the baby into the family's routines and rituals. It can be helpful to do this far enough in advance so the change can happen gradually. Families might consider

- Adding pictures of the baby to family pictures around the house

- Talking with siblings about what the baby might be doing at particular times of the day

- Praying for the baby during nightly prayers with siblings or during family prayer time

- Including the baby in special holiday rituals, such as having siblings pick out a special Halloween bib or a new Christmas tree ornament for the baby

Integrating a new member into any family can create changes in families' routines. For many, daily routines will need to be adapted following the baby's discharge from the hospital. Incorporating the baby's caregiving needs into families' regular routines can take time, trial and error, and patience. Families can become frustrated when they see that what works well in one situation may not work in another. They may need information on where to locate support and assistance with this issue after the baby has been discharged.

Young siblings may have favorite books and lullaby CDs that have become a regular part of their bedtime routine. Older siblings may have favorite books they enjoy reading over and over, as well as favorite music, which they often play at home and the baby may hear on a regular basis. Siblings may want to share some of these favorites with the baby prior to discharge. Sharing young siblings' items can help integrate the baby into siblings' bedtime routine. Older siblings can read favorite books, or even homework assignments, to the baby and let the baby listen to their favorite music as well. Families should be reminded not to leave siblings' books or CDs at the hospital, as siblings can become upset if their items are lost or misplaced. Families should also continue to monitor siblings' activities with the baby to ensure that the baby is not being overstimulated.

SAFETY ISSUES FOR SIBLINGS AND THE BABY

As part of the discharge process, basic safety and infection control issues should be discussed with families. Depending on the baby's medical needs, issues such as siblings' immunizations, normal childhood illnesses, and attendance at center-based child care or preschool may need to be considered. It can also be helpful to share basic safety information with siblings, such as hand washing, infection control, holding the baby, and the baby's sleeping positions.

Families should also consider environmental safety issues, especially when a young sibling will be sharing a room with the baby following discharge. Families need to be aware of the possibility of young siblings getting into the baby's crib. Some siblings can be very creative and stack an assortment of items that allows them to climb into the crib to visit the baby. Families should also be aware of siblings' access to items they can throw into the crib or push between the bars to share with the baby. Families may need to check on the sibling and baby frequently, as well as consider investing in a baby monitor.

Babies who have been hospitalized for an extended period may have rolling or scooting mobility by the time they are discharged. Family members, including siblings, may need information on ways to child proof their home so it is not only safe for the baby upon discharge, but also as the baby develops. Some possessions of older siblings can present aspiration risks for the baby. Siblings may need to find places where they can play, do homework, and keep their possessions away from the baby.

Before the baby's discharge, a safe place should be found for the baby's medications to help prevent accidental ingestion by siblings or the baby. It is also important to discuss child-resistant packaging with parents. Some parents may believe this means that all children are unable to open the container; therefore, they do not need to be as careful where they keep the medicine. If parents are to draw up or set out a day's worth of medication, it is important that it be kept in a safe place and out of reach of climbing siblings as well.

CONCLUSION

The anticipated discharge of a baby from the hospital can be an exciting experience for the entire family. Different siblings can have different interest levels in participating in this process and should be supported in their decision as often as possible. As interested, they can benefit from opportunities to help get ready for the baby at home, as well as learn aspects of the baby's care and important safety information. These opportunities can help them to feel a part of this important family event.

The Baby Comes Home

Including Big Brothers and Sisters

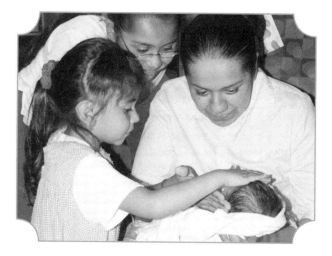

When the baby comes home from the hospital, it is beneficial for the family to spend time together as a unit. Some families may consider having siblings stay with extended family or family friends until the baby is settled in the home environment; however, exclusion from this important family event can be difficult for siblings to understand, and they may feel replaced or forgotten. It might be better to have a familiar, consistent caregiver support and care for siblings at home during this time.

BABY'S TRANSITION INTO THE HOME ENVIRONMENT

The transition or adjustment period after the baby is home can be challenging for many families. They are adjusting to caring for the baby without the consistent support they had in the hospital and must now combine this with caring for siblings and completing household and job responsibilities. Families may need continued assistance as they support the baby's transition into the home environment. Resolving the baby's health care issues can take time and may not always be a smooth process. Maroney (1995), a NICU nurse and mother of a premature daughter, reported that the baby's homecoming can be a bigger adjustment than anticipated, and there may be little time and energy available for siblings. VandenBerg (1999) discussed that premature babies can be disorganized for an extended time following discharge and can easily be overstimulated. Parents may need assistance and support adapting the home environment to meet these challenges.

Mr. and Mrs. Marks took their premature baby, Jonah, home from the NICU a few weeks before his anticipated due date. His 3-year-old sister, Amy, was excited that he was home. She talked to Jonah while Mrs. Marks fed him, and after he ate, Amy pushed him in his new swing. Mrs. Marks began to notice that Jonah was eating less than he had in the hospital, was spitting up during and following his feedings, and was beginning to show an increase in overstimulation cues. She explained to Amy that when Jonah ate, it was his special time with Mommy and that afterward he needed to be still and have quiet time to help the milk stay in his tummy. She reminded Amy that bedtime was her special time with Mommy and that they would be able to read stories and snuggle together then.

The D'Amico children, Sofia, Mario, and Anna, ages 5, 8, and 13, were excited and happy that their new baby sister, Tessa, was home after an extended stay in the hospital. Sofia expected that she would continue to spend special time with her momma after school time, but when this did not happen, she became angry and began to slam doors and play the television loudly. When Mario and Anna came home from school, they blasted their music to hear it over the television, and at times their house became like Grand Central Station as friends called and came by.

Mr. and Mrs. D'Amico noticed that Tessa became more disorganized after her siblings came home from school. She showed increased overstimulation cues such as agitation, fussiness, back arching, gaze aversion, finger splaying, and hiccups. After meeting with some of her physicians, they decided to put Tessa in their room upstairs after school, which was quieter, and established a new family rule that friends visiting after school were to stay downstairs. They also contacted the local high school and found a student who required community service hours for graduation and was interested in a career with children to spend time with Sofia after school. In addition, they invested in headphones for their older children to quietly listen to music.

SIBLING COPING ISSUES

Siblings can be overwhelmed by the number of visitors who come to see the baby at home. Young siblings who have not seen some of these individuals recently may view them as strangers because they do not remember them from past visits. They can also have difficulty as visitors arrive with gifts for the baby and not for them.

Tip for Families

Having a supply of small gifts on hand for young siblings can help them feel remembered when numerous visitors arrive with gifts for the baby.

Some visitors can be supportive for older siblings, especially when parents' time and attention are focused on the baby, although other visitors may need gentle reminders that siblings need to be acknowledged as well as the baby. Siblings, however, can become annoyed when visitors pinch them on the cheek, pat them on the head, or tell them how much they have grown. They can grow tired of answering questions and comments such as "Aren't you glad the baby is home?" and "You are such a great helper for your mom and dad." In some cases, siblings may need assistance to cope with this situation or have time away from visitors built into their schedule.

In some families, siblings' developmental concerns can easily but unintentionally be pushed aside when the baby comes home. With only so many hours in the day, families can be stretched just meeting the baby's needs.

Families may need to identify individuals who can assist siblings with developmental concerns until some of the baby's issues are resolved.

Older Infant and Toddler Siblings

Older infant and toddler siblings are extremely dependent on their parents and can have difficulty sharing their parents' time and attention with the new baby. They may need extra cuddling and reassurance as they cope with the addition of the baby to the home environment. They may begin to cling to their parents more and have increased difficulty separating from them even in environments where this has not been an issue.

The baby's feeding times can also be troublesome for these siblings. Some may still be nursing or be using a bottle on a regular basis or only at specific times of the day. If they have recently been weaned, they may feel that the baby has usurped their position. Providing extra snuggle time with Mommy or another special adult during or following the baby's feedings may help siblings cope with negative feelings.

Preschool Siblings

Although many preschool siblings have adjusted to being a big brother or sister by the time the baby is discharged, having the baby at home can be very different from visiting the baby in the hospital. Preschool siblings may have difficulty coping as the focus of family life at home increasingly shifts toward the baby. They may attempt to attract the family's attention away from the baby and back to themselves. They may also try to attract attention in other environments, such as preschool or center-based child care, so it can be helpful to inform teachers and other appropriate adults about the baby's homecoming.

Some babies who have been hospitalized in the NICU tend to become easily overstimulated, which can be a difficult issue for preschool siblings who may be very excited that the baby is finally home and want to be near the baby. They may need to learn ways to interact without overstimulating the baby in this new environment. Babies who can tolerate this stimulation often enjoy observing and listening to the commotion and chaos these siblings can cause around them. Interaction with preschool siblings, as well as other siblings, can also have a positive impact on the baby's development.

School-Age Siblings

School-age siblings are often excited that the baby is home from the hospital and can be enthusiastic about helping with caregiving issues; however, as time progresses and the newness of having the baby at home begins to wear off, this can change. The baby may require even more of the family's time and energy at home than it did in the hospital, which can make some siblings begin to feel as if the baby has taken over their home, parents, and possibly their place in the family. Parents can respond to this by creating a baby-free space for siblings, building individual time with siblings into the family routine as often as possible, and trying to ensure that the baby's needs are not continuously placed before the siblings.

This may be the first time that friends of school-age siblings have had an opportunity to see the baby other than in photographs. Siblings may need assistance and support on ways to respond to their friends' questions and reactions to the baby, such as "Why does your baby have to go to the doctor all the time? Isn't he well yet?" or "Why does your baby cry and spit up so much? My baby sister didn't do that," or "She's so teeny tiny!" They may also need assistance on how to share information positively with their friends about some of the baby's specific issues, such as the importance of hand washing and friends' not visiting when they are sick.

Preteen and Adolescent Siblings

Preteen and adolescent siblings also tend to get excited when the baby comes home and are often interested in participating in aspects of the baby's care; however, their involvement with friends, school, and extracurricular activities may limit their ability to participate on a regular basis. Many older siblings enjoy entertainment through electronics, such as CD players, televisions, DVDs, and video games, which can overstimulate the baby if played loudly. Headphones can be used with these items, but in addition to making it more difficult to share entertainment, headphones can isolate the preteen or adolescent from the rest of the family if used frequently. Also, playing headphones loudly for long periods may lead to hearing loss.

As with school-age siblings, this may be the first time that friends of preteen and adolescent siblings have seen the baby other than in pictures. Siblings may need assistance with sharing information about the baby, as well as how to respond to any negative comments. In some cases, they may not receive any comments, which can be difficult for them as well.

INFECTION CONTROL AND SAFETY ISSUES

Safety information should be shared with siblings after the baby is home. They may need to know what they can do independently with the baby and when they should ask for assistance. Providing siblings with a general list of times when they should ask for help may prevent them from attempting to imitate how they have seen others care for the baby. The list might include

- Picking up the baby
- Giving the baby anything to eat or drink
- Changing the baby's diapers or clothes
- Sharing toys with the baby

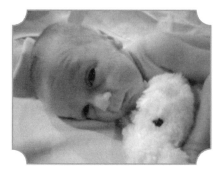

The list should be short and simple so that siblings can remember it easily. Siblings might also be informed about what they can do independently with the baby. These activities can vary and will depend on the siblings' developmental level, the baby's developmental and medical issues, and the parents' comfort level.

Hand Washing

Hand washing continues to be important after the baby is home. There are a variety of ways families can help facilitate sibling hand washing. One is to provide a stable step stool for young siblings who are unable to reach the sink, which can also help increase their sense of independence and reduce chances of them climbing on unsafe drawers or the toilet to reach it. Another way to facilitate hand washing is to provide fun soaps in different shapes, colors, or scents, as well as special towels, which might also keep siblings from drying their hands on their clothes. Young siblings may enjoy being part of the baby's germ patrol by reminding visitors to wash their hands before they touch the baby or not to get close to the baby when they are sick. Siblings may also be interested in helping to make and decorate safety signs, such as "Please wash your hands" to hang near the baby's crib, or "I am tiny and trying to stay well, so please be careful when you cough and sneeze" for the stroller. Older siblings may enjoy using the computer to print out a list of hand washing steps for visitors. They may wish to make a sign for the front door instructing visitors on the importance of infection control, including hand washing.

Tip for Families

Adults in the household should be good role models for siblings and other children around the baby when it comes to hand washing.

Medications

When the baby needs medication at home, families need to consider siblings' and the baby's safety. Medication should be purchased in child-resistant packaging and stored out of children's reach and climbing range. Parents also need to consider medication safety issues when visitors are in their home. These visitors may have medication with them, and they may not always be cognizant of safety issues.

FOLLOW-UP APPOINTMENTS

Babies who have been hospitalized often have follow-up outpatient appointments after discharge. The number and types of these appointments can vary depending on the baby's diagnosis and hospital experience. Ritchie (2002) reported that some appointments may be at clinics connected with the hospital but, because of the regionalization of NICUs, may not always be close to the family's home. This can pose scheduling or financial difficulties for some families.

Siblings may want to be included in the baby's outpatient appointments. Their need for information about the baby's health and medical care does not end just because the baby is home. They may have concerns about the number of appointments, especially those that take place near the hospital. They may also worry that the baby's health is deteriorating and that the baby will need to be rehospitalized. Being able to discuss some of these issues with their family, as well as members of the baby's health care team, can be beneficial for siblings.

Tip for Families

It is important for siblings to be acknowledged during follow-up appointments. If they are excluded from conversations, they can begin to feel as if they are invisible or that their issues are not important.

In some families, siblings may not have a choice about being included in follow-up appointments. Because of the baby's medical bills, some families may be unable to afford the additional cost of child care, so they may have to take young siblings with them. Babies who have been hospitalized can be more susceptible to infections, so the family may need to wait in an exam room instead of the regular waiting room where there may be toys. Because young siblings may have a hard time sitting still if the wait is long, families should be encouraged to bring a few toys and activities to help keep the baby and siblings occupied. In other cases, appointments may be scheduled around siblings' routines, particularly school, making it difficult for siblings to be involved and more stressful for families when appointments are delayed or take longer than expected.

EMERGENCY ISSUES

In many hospitals, families are provided with CPR instruction before the baby's discharge from the NICU. The American Academy of Pediatrics (1998) recommended that families' competence with infant CPR be demonstrated before the discharge. The chance of an emergency can depend on many issues, some being the baby's diagnosis, medical course, or the family's ability to care for the baby at home. If an emergency occurs, parents can be frightened and overwhelmed as they try to recall what they were taught at the hospital. They also may not have enough time or energy to support siblings during this experience. Families should consider this issue before an emergency occurs and formulate a plan that includes ways for siblings to help during the emergency, as well as caregivers to contact to provide care for siblings.

Siblings can be involved in preparations for an emergency situation. For example, families need to ensure that their home address is clearly visible, day and night, so that paramedics and other emergency workers, as well as home health care staff, can locate the home easily. Gavin (2004) stated that house numbers should be clearly visible from the street. This can be made into a family project and can help reinforce the family's address for siblings. Families may also want to consider taking young siblings on a field trip to the local fire station. This can allow them to see some of the emergency vehicles up close in a nonemergency situation, and siblings can possibly meet some of the paramedics and firefighters who might respond to an emergency situation at their home. It also provides families with an opportunity to share information about the baby's medical needs with the fire station staff before an emergency occurs.

Some siblings may be able to play a role in an emergency situation whereas others may not. The degree of siblings' involvement will vary according to their developmental level and coping skills. Some siblings may be able to talk with an emergency medical services (EMS) or 911 operator while their parents are dealing with the baby's emergency situation. Gavin (2004) discussed how siblings may need assistance in understanding when they should call 911 and when they should not and that they should be instructed not to hang up until they are told by the operator. She also recommended role-playing with siblings so they can practice their skills before an emergency occurs and practice answering questions that an EMS or 911 operator might ask. This also allows parents to see if siblings have an accurate recall of the information they may need to provide. Gavin also suggested creating an information sheet for children to read in an emergency situation. If the emergency occurs somewhere other than the family's home, siblings should be reminded to give the address and telephone number of their actual location.

Another role siblings may have in an emergency situation is waiting for the ambulance or other emergency vehicles to arrive. If they wait at the curb, they should be reminded not to stand in the street to flag down any vehicles or individuals, as sometimes family rules can be forgotten in a crisis situation. Siblings can also gather supplies their parents and the baby may need at the hospital, such as medical information and a change of clothes.

READMISSION TO THE NICU

Babies who have been hospitalized in the NICU can be at great risk for rehospitalization on the basis of their diagnosis. Escobar et al. (1999) stated that babies who were premature tended to be at risk for rehospitalization. Carbonell-Estrany et al. (2000) reported that premature babies with chronic lung disease (CLD) had a higher risk of being rehospitalized for respiratory syncytial virus. Premature babies diagnosed with CLD who required oxygen at 36 weeks and premature babies with CLD who needed oxygen at home tended to be rehospitalized more frequently (Elder, Hagan, Evans, Benninger, & French, 1999; Lamarche-Vadel et al., 2004).

Individual characteristics of the baby and family may also factor into the premature baby's risk for rehospitalization. Elder et al. (1999), Escobar et al. (1999), and Escobar et al. (2005) reported that boys are more likely to be readmitted than girls. Carbonell-Estrany et al. (2000) and Lamarche-Vadel et al. (2004) reported that having siblings can increase the potential for re-hospitalization. Lower socioeconomic status and mothers who smoke are other risk factors for the baby's rehospitalization.

Siblings' Concerns

The baby's rehospitalization can be difficult for the entire family. Parents may believe they have failed in providing adequate care for the baby, while siblings may fear that the baby will die or that they have somehow caused the baby to be rehospitalized. Siblings may have questions about the baby returning to the hospital, and some of their fears and concerns from the initial hospitalization may resurface. They may need follow-up support during this time to ensure they have a clear understanding of why the baby was readmitted. Families may also need support with this issue and assistance in contacting the child life specialist or social worker for the unit where the baby was admitted.

Support for Siblings

When the baby is rehospitalized, siblings' information and support needs often increase. Information about the baby's rehospitalization should be aimed at siblings' developmental level and shared in a way that helps clear up misconceptions or misunderstandings and encourages them to express their questions and concerns. Siblings can also benefit from opportunities to participate in the baby's rehospitalization, such as visiting the baby in the new unit and meeting members of the new health care team.

During this time, it can be helpful to utilize familiar, consistent care-givers and continue as many family routines as possible. Now that the baby has become part of the home routine, parents may feel less comfortable about leaving the baby at the hospital without their support. As a result, siblings may be separated even more from their parents during the baby's re-hospitalizations.

The Emergency Center and Siblings

Babies who have been hospitalized in the NICU can become sick very quickly, and trips to the emergency center at a nearby hospital may be necessary. An inability to locate child care on such short notice may require siblings to accompany their parents and the baby. Parents should be aware of what siblings might see or hear while waiting in the hospital emergency center that could frighten or confuse them. Many children's hospitals have child life specialists working in their emergency centers who are trained to help children understand and cope with their emergency center experience. They may be able to assist siblings and act as a resource for families as well.

CONCLUSION

The baby's homecoming from the hospital is often a time of transition for many families. Sharing information with siblings and providing them with opportunities to have a role in this process has the potential to help them to have a more positive adjustment to the addition of the baby in their home environment. Families can often benefit from information on ways to support siblings and help them cope throughout this process.

12

Understanding the Baby's Death

Support for Siblings

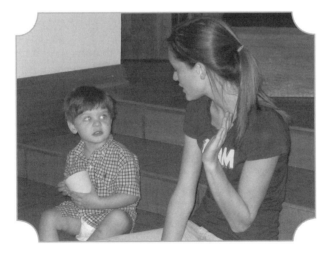

The majority of babies in the NICU will recover and go home with their families to live what is hoped will be a long, happy life. Occasionally, however, a baby dies, either in the hospital, in a hospice, or at home. This can be a devastating experience for the baby's entire family, including siblings. As the baby's condition deteriorates, information should be shared with siblings to allow them to begin the process of anticipating the baby's death. When information is not shared, siblings may be taken by surprise, even if the baby has been hospitalized for an extended time.

Mahon and Page (1995) reported that if the sibling's death is preceded by an extended illness, children tend to be surprised when the death occurs because they were often not aware of the seriousness of the diagnosis. On the other hand, as Mahon (1994) reported, when children are aware of the seriousness of their sibling's condition, they may believe it will improve as it has in the past, and, therefore, the sibling's death can easily take them by surprise as well.

DNR STATUS AND TREATMENT WITHDRAWAL

Families can face a myriad of issues when confronted with the decision of do-not-resuscitate (DNR) or removal of life support. These issues can be especially difficult to explain to siblings, and families may request assistance and support. When explaining the decision of DNR, it can be helpful to discuss some of the options that have been tried in the past and were unsuccessful. Options that will continue to be provided should be emphasized rather than those that will not, such as resuscitation. Siblings who have concerns about the amount of pain the baby might experience should be assured that the health care team will do all it can to make sure that the baby is not in pain.

When the decision is made to remove life support, families may need assistance with sibling issues. Whenever possible, families should be informed about the length of time that can be anticipated for the baby to die following the removal of life support. This information can help them make the most appropriate decision for their family about including their children in this process and also allows them to either prepare siblings for participation or arrange for child care if needed. McHaffie, Lyon, and Fowlie (2001) interviewed families that had discussed treatment limitations with their baby's medical team several months after their baby had died. They reported that several of these families had expected that their baby would die immediately or soon after life support was removed, but when the baby lingered on, some of these families began to reevaluate their decision. The interviewers also reported that after life support was withdrawn, families expressed anguish and distress over the changes the baby went through as he or she died. Parents should be prepared for these changes not only for their sake but so that they can also explain them to siblings and other family members. It should be noted that the increase in parental distress may cause an increase in sibling distress.

SIBLING GRIEF

Many siblings, even very young ones, develop a loving relationship with the baby and will grieve as the rest of their family will when the baby dies. Including siblings in the family's mourning experiences can help reduce feelings of isolation as well as reduce misunderstandings. Siblings grieve as members of their family, and the way their family copes can affect the way they cope. Hames (2003) and Monroe and Kraus (1996) stated that children can utilize the adults in their family as role models for appropriate grief behavior and coping.

Each child is a unique individual and responds to death differently, even children from the same family. Some issues that can affect how siblings cope with the baby's death include their developmental level, temperament, prior experiences with death, coping styles, the availability of support systems, the accuracy and timing of information provided about the baby's death, and opportunities to participate in the family's mourning process and experiences.

Older Infant and Toddler Siblings

Older infant and toddler siblings are often able to recognize changes in family members' emotions, such as increased sadness and grief when a loved one dies. They can also recognize changes in their daily routines, such as no longer being left with a familiar caregiver while their parents visit the baby in the NICU. Hames (2003) reported that infants may cry more and show changes in their eating and sleeping habits. She also claimed that toddlers may show regression, have increased temper tantrums, cling to familiar caregivers, have intensified separation anxiety, and possibly believe they caused the baby's death and have the power to bring the baby back to life. Frequent accurate explanations in simple language can help toddlers understand the situation and provide reassurance that they will continue to be cared for.

Zhen, age 2, was with her family as her baby brother died in a hospice setting. She saw her parents cry and grieve for hours. The next week, she had difficulty saying good-bye to her mother at center-based child care, began having intense temper tantrums, and refused to go to sleep at night.

Preschool Siblings

Preschool siblings can also recognize changes in family members' emotions and in their daily routines that may signify that something important has happened in their family. They tend to benefit from developmentally appropriate information about the baby's death, although families should not be made to feel guilty if they need time to process the information beforehand or if sharing information with children is not in line with their cultural or religious beliefs. Preschool siblings have a tendency to interpret explanations literally and can easily misinterpret euphemisms that families might use when discussing the baby's death. Rubel (2005) reported that preschoolers tend to benefit from explanations that refer to the physical body, such as the body is not working or a specific part of the body is not working.

Preschoolers also tend to view death as a temporary separation. Christ (2000), Rubel (2005), and Zeitlin (2001) reported that these siblings often have difficulty understanding the permanence of death. They may believe that the baby will come back to life, which can affect how they may cope with the baby's death as well as the types of questions they might ask. Christ also stated that preschoolers tend to ask repetitive questions after the death of a loved one. These questions can often help them process and better understand the experience and are not just a way to drive parents and other adults crazy.

The pattern of preschool siblings' grief can be different from that of adults. Zeitlin (2001) discussed that children can grieve for short periods while continuing with aspects of their daily routines. She explained that this is a way for them to protect themselves from some of the intense emotions they might experience. Because of this, adults can mistakenly believe that the baby's death has not affected them. Preschool siblings may also combine aspects of death and dying in their play and artwork.

Colin, age 3, was with his family when his baby brother died in the NICU. Over the next several weeks, Colin's family observed that he tended to grieve for his brother for brief periods and then easily returned to his play. They mistakenly assumed that Colin did not care that his baby brother had died.

Charlotte returned to preschool a week after her baby sister had died in the NICU. She spent much of her first weeks back in preschool in the housekeeping corner with the baby dolls, playing "the baby has died."

Preschool siblings can believe that they have somehow caused the baby to die. Zeitlin (2001) reported that this belief is not something that siblings are usually able to articulate and share with their family.

Three-year-old Larissa picked out a special balloon to take to her baby brother in the hospital but decided instead to take it home and keep it in her room.

A few days later, the baby was diagnosed with an infection and quickly died. Larissa was convinced that her baby brother died because she had not given him the balloon. She became quieter than usual, and her parents assumed she was grieving.

Rasheed was tired of all the time his parents were spending at the hospital with his baby sister. He wished that his dad could coach his soccer team, go to his games, and kick the soccer ball with him after supper like he used to. Several days later, the baby's condition worsened, and she died. Rasheed believed that he caused his baby sister to die because he wanted to play soccer with his dad and decided to punish himself by not playing soccer. Rasheed's grieving parents, however, assumed he was not playing soccer because he was grieving as well.

After their experience with the baby's death, preschool siblings may have difficulty with their own encounters with health care. Their perception may be that when people are sick, they go to the hospital where they die. These siblings will need appropriate preparation, support, and follow-up for future health care experiences, especially those that include hospitalization and emergency room visits.

School-Age Siblings

School-age siblings' understanding of death and dying may be more mature than that of younger siblings, but they can continue to have misconceptions. Rubel (2005) reported that school-age children are better able to understand the permanence of death but can still have difficulty discussing aspects of it. Although they tend to benefit from receiving accurate information in a timely fashion, it may not always be necessary to share all the details. In addition, they can still often misunderstand euphemisms commonly used by adults. Pettle and Britten (1995) stated that school-age children who are interested in what happens to the body after death may ask questions about subjects such as the morgue, autopsies, or organ donation. They may have picked up these topics from adult conversations or from movies or television.

Jeannie, age 7, was with her family when her baby sister died in a hospice setting. After the baby's death, the family spent time together saying good-bye to the baby. After several hours, they were ready to go home. Jeannie knew they would not be returning and asked questions about what would happen to her baby sister. The social worker shared basic information with Jeannie about what would happen to the baby's body and then discussed funeral homes with her parents.

He also informed Jeannie's parents that she might continue to ask questions about what would happen to the baby and provided referrals for support.

Nine-year-old Simone was with her family when her baby brother died in the NICU. An avid fan of television medical shows, she was aware that after people died they went to the morgue and often had an autopsy, although she did not have a clear understanding of what either meant. After saying good-bye to her brother, she began to ask numerous questions about the morgue, autopsies, and organ donation. This was more than her grieving parents could handle.

With permission from Simone's parents, the baby's bedside nurse assisted Simone with some of her questions and concerns using developmentally appropriate language. They discussed that the baby would go to the hospital's morgue, which was in the basement, after the family left the hospital. An autopsy, which would determine why the baby died, was not needed because they already knew why he had died. The nurse also told Simone that because her baby brother had had a severe infection, organ donation would not be possible, but that this was an important issue for her to bring up.

The nurse went on to explain that when Simone's family made a decision about a funeral home, people from its staff would pick up the baby's body from the morgue at the hospital. They would then take it to the funeral home and prepare it for whatever type of funeral her family had chosen. The most important thing for her to remember was that the baby's body would always be well cared for.

School-age siblings may need to take breaks in the grieving process if it becomes too intense for them. Rubel (2005) discussed that school-age children can go from showing extreme emotions to acting as if nothing has happened. Rubel also reported that siblings may have difficulty sleeping, experience nightmares, have difficulty concentrating, be more aggressive, and possibly believe they have caused their loved one to die.

One night during his bedtime prayers, 6-year-old Ramon prayed that his baby brother would go away for a while so that his parents could spend time with him like they did before the baby was born. The next day, the baby unexpectedly died. Ramon was afraid to tell his parents what he had done for fear they would blame him for the baby's death.

Renee, age 8, decided to go on a long weekend trip to the beach with her best friend's family rather than visit her baby sister in the NICU. While she was away, her baby sister took a turn for the worse and died. When Renee re-

turned, her parents told her the terrible news. Renee believed that if she had decided not to go on the trip, her baby sister might still be alive. She discussed her concern with her grandmother, who repeatedly reassured her that no one was responsible for the baby's death.

After the baby's death, school-age siblings, like preschool siblings, may view the hospital as a place where people die and may have difficulty with future health care experiences. They, too, will need to receive appropriate preparation, support, and follow-up.

Siblings may also find it difficult to concentrate in school following the baby's death, and parents who are grieving may not be as available to provide support and guidance during homework and study time. When siblings' teachers are made aware of the situation, they can help support them upon their return to school and can also share information with parents about their coping issues. Compassionate Friends (2003) reported that teachers can help with the way classmates interact with the grieving sibling. These children may not know what to do or say and so may say nothing at all. This can send an upsetting message to siblings that their classmates do not care about them or their situation.

Preteen Siblings

The preteen years tend to be a time of great change. Preteens not only gain information about death and dying issues from their family but also from peers; other adults in their environment; and media such as books, magazines, and especially television and movies. Preteen siblings can benefit from opportunities to grieve on their own timetable. There will be times when they request a great deal of information and times when they do not want to discuss the baby at all. There will also be times when they want information but do not know how to ask for it. Even though their understanding of death and dying is approaching an adult level, preteens continue to need a great amount of support and comfort but may sometimes have difficulty articulating this need. They may also be reluctant to grieve or express their emotions in front of others.

Sarah and Emily, ages 10 and 12 years old, were with their family in the NICU as their baby brother died. In the days and weeks following the baby's death, Sarah had numerous questions about the baby's death and shared memories of her visits to the NICU with others. Emily, who grieved differently, asked very few questions about the baby's death and did not want to talk about him in front of others.

Preteen siblings may also have difficulty concentrating in school or can show a lack of interest in schoolwork following the baby's death. For some preteens, however, school can be a comforting part of their regular routine. Christ (2000) discussed that preteens may use school and other activities as a diversion from their grief. In addition, death, dying, and coping issues may show up in some of their schoolwork, such as writing and art projects, and even in doodles in the margins of their notebooks. It can be beneficial for families to communicate with siblings' teachers before and following the baby's death, even if it occurs during a school holiday. Santoro and Bennett-Santoro (n.d.) suggested that siblings and their parents write a letter to siblings' teachers that not only communicates information about their brother's or sister's death but also provides information about coping techniques that have been successful for the siblings and any additional support that may be needed. Families may decide to mail the letter to siblings' teachers and other school personnel or arrange a meeting with teachers, parents, and siblings.

Theresa Rae's baby sister recently died at home following an extended NICU hospitalization. After consulting with Theresa Rae (age 11), her mother contacted the school and informed them about the baby's death. When she returned to school, Theresa Rae had difficulty concentrating and spent large amounts of time staring off into space and doodling in the margins of her notebook. Consequently, her grades began to fall. Theresa Rae, her mother, and some of her teachers met to discuss possible ways to help her cope during school and complete her schoolwork.

Adolescent Siblings

The teenage years continue to be a time of great change. Busch and Kimble (2001) reported that even though adolescents have developed an adult-level understanding of death, they can lack the maturity, coping skills, and life experiences to help them deal with this experience. Their views of death can be influenced by family, cultural, and religious beliefs, as well as what they have seen in movies and on television and what they have discussed with their friends. For some teens, this may be their first experience with the death of a loved one, and they can need assistance and support from their family and other important adults in their life. Some adolescents may have difficulty sharing their questions, concerns, or feelings regarding the baby's death. Rubel (2005) suggested that although friends can provide some support, adults are often more effective in providing support and honest information about death and dying issues.

Before and after the baby's death, some adolescents, like some pre-teens, may find it difficult to concentrate in school or be less interested in schoolwork. If they have missed school during this time, they may also have difficulty completing makeup work. Rubel (2005) discussed that grieving adolescents may need continued support at school even if their grades are not dropping. For some adolescents, school can be a respite from the grief at home. Compassionate Friends (2003) reported that school routines can provide comforting normalcy when life at home may be chaotic following the death of a family member.

Ian and Sean, age 13 and 16 years old, were with their family as their baby sister died in a hospice setting. After consulting with the boys, their mother contacted the counselor at their school to inform her that the baby had died. The following week, when the boys returned to school, their responses were different. Ian continued to do very well and utilized school as an escape from the grief at home. Sean, on the other hand, had difficulty concentrating and often failed to get his assignments in on time. Both boys continued to meet on a periodic basis with the school counselor.

ADDRESSING SIBLINGS' NEEDS

Parents may need assistance in supporting their children before and after the baby's death. Ayyash-Abdo (2001) reported that parents may not be aware of their children's level of understanding of death and dying issues and, because they are often actively grieving themselves, may need time to process information before they can share it with their children. There are a variety of professionals, such as child life specialists, social workers, and possibly psychologists and psychiatrists, who are available to assist and support parents with these issues. Families can also use siblings' primary pediatrician as a resource. The American Academy of Pediatrics (2000) discussed that the primary pediatrician has a history with the family, as well as knowledge of the family's medical background and certain psychosocial issues, and can often be a source of information for parents on death and dying issues.

Some families can benefit from utilizing an extended family member, family friend, or other supportive individual to assist grieving parents as they support siblings with death and dying issues. They can often provide assistance in this role long after the family has left the hospital or hospice. Wilson (2001) mentioned that these individuals may also be a source of support for siblings who have difficulty discussing the baby's death with their parents.

Talking with Siblings About the Baby's Death

Talking with their children about the baby's death or imminent death can be one of the most challenging aspects of this experience for many parents. Wilson (2001) discussed the difficulty grieving families can have with providing accurate information and answering their children's questions following a miscarriage or the death of a baby. Their past experiences with death and dying issues as well as the family's cultural background and religious beliefs can influence what they are comfortable discussing with their children. Different members of the same family can have different beliefs and opinions on this issue. Some may believe that the best way to help siblings through this experience is by not informing them of the baby's death. Others may believe that sharing information with siblings is beneficial but may be unsure how, especially when they are grieving themselves.

Table 3.   Misleading euphemisms used to describe the baby's death to children

Euphemisms	Misinterpretations
The baby went to sleep. The baby is sleeping.	I might die the next time I go to sleep. I am never going to sleep again.
The baby went on a trip.	Daddy's going on a trip. Will he die like the baby did?
The baby went away.	Will I be sent away, too?
The good die young.	If I am good, I will die, too, so I'm going to be bad.
The baby passed on. The baby passed.	Where did the baby pass to?
We lost the baby.	Why is no one looking for the baby? What will happen if I am lost? Would anyone look for me?
The baby is in a better place.	What's wrong with this place? We are still here.
The baby died because he was sick.	Mommy has a headache, and Daddy has a tummy ache. Are they going to die?
The baby died because he was in the hospital.	I fell off the slide and broke my arm. Daddy took me to the hospital to get it fixed. Am I going to die?
The baby kicked the bucket.	Is the baby in a bucket? Is someone kicking the baby?
The baby is your guardian angel. The baby is living on a cloud with the angels.	Will airplanes hit the baby when they fly through the clouds? Can we see the baby the next time we ride on an airplane and fly above the clouds?

God took the baby to live with him.
  The baby went to live with God.
  God took the baby.
  It's God's will.
	Will God take me next?
	Will God take Mommy and Daddy to live with him next and leave me here all by myself?

God never gives us more than we can handle.	Why does God want to hold the baby's hand?
We are not given more than we can bear.	Is a bear going to hurt the baby? Will the bear hurt me next?
It was a blessing.	Would it be a blessing if I died, too?

As they discuss the death of a loved one, adults may use euphemisms that children can easily misunderstand. Table 3 provides examples of these euphemisms, as well as some of the ways siblings can misunderstand them. Because children tend to interpret information literally, euphemisms may leave siblings with an entirely different understanding from what the speaker intended. Zeitlin (2001) recommended avoiding euphemisms with children, but this can be difficult for families that cannot bring themselves to say "The baby is going to die" or "The baby died." Families should also be aware of how others may have discussed the baby's death with siblings.

Other factors to keep in mind when speaking with siblings include using developmentally appropriate language, providing information in a timely manner, and using an atmosphere of open communication. Pettle and Britten (1995) reported that adults can overestimate the amount of information children have understood about the death of a loved one. It can therefore be helpful to encourage siblings to share their understanding of the baby's death and the information they have received.

Parents with children at different developmental levels may want to share information about the baby's death as a family unit. Doing so can provide an atmosphere of love and support in which siblings can also be a source of support and information for each other.

Saying Good-bye to the Health Care Team

After the baby has died and before the family leaves the hospital or hospice, siblings may want to say good-bye to members of the baby's health care team who have become special to them. Parents who are grieving can sometimes overlook this possibility. If caregivers are not available, siblings may wish to leave a note or drawing for them. If the family's departure leaves no time for this, siblings can mail their note or drawing to the hospital or hospice. After the baby has died, families may need time before they are able to return to the hospital or hospice setting (e.g., to see other babies). Because of this, siblings may or may not have opportunities to see these special caregivers again. Siblings may also want to say good-bye to members of other families they have met at the NICU or hospice.

CEREMONIES AND RITUALS FOR THE BABY

Families may have a variety of questions and concerns about ways to include siblings in ceremonies and rituals related to the baby's death. Adult family members may never have attended these ceremonies as children and can be unsure if and how to include their own children, as well as how to help them through this experience. Siblings grieve as members of their family, and their involvement in these ceremonies and rituals can be a positive experience. Stuber and Mesrkhani (2001) suggested that sibling participation should be a joint decision between parents and the child, whereas Barrett and Schuurman (2000), Busch and Kimble (2001), DeMaso, Meyer, and Beasley (1997),

Holland (2004), Pettle and Britten (1995), and Rubel (2005) recommended giving children a choice about attending the funeral service. These ceremonies and rituals can give family and friends a chance to gather together and support one another as they share memories of the baby. When siblings are not given an opportunity to attend, they can feel separated and alone at a time when they need the comfort and support of their family the most.

Siblings' participation in family mourning ceremonies or private family good-bye gatherings can provide memories for parents to share when discussing the baby's death with siblings, such as "Remember when we went to the baby's funeral? We saw all the people who were there to say good-bye to the baby," or "Our baby died and is in heaven. Remember when we said the special prayers at his grave and you let the balloons go? They went up very high, didn't they?" or "Remember when we went to the baby's grave and took the pretty flowers?"

How and when families are comfortable including siblings in ceremonies for the baby will vary from child to child and family to family and may be influenced by the sibling's developmental level and temperament, as well as the family's support systems and cultural and religious beliefs. Some families are comfortable with all siblings, even very young ones, attending these ceremonies, while others are not. Some family members, however, may disagree with the parents' decision about including siblings. Parents may overhear negative comments and begin to question whether they made the right decision for their children and family. They may need assistance and support from the health care team with this issue, especially if they are not receiving any from their family or friends.

Preparing Siblings for Ceremonies and Rituals

For many siblings, this may be their first experience attending a funeral service. The American Academy of Pediatrics (2000), Barrett and Schuurman (2000), Busch and Kimble (2001), Holland (2004), Monroe and Kraus (1996), Pettle and Britten (1995), and Rubel (2005) recommended that siblings be prepared before attending the funeral service. Preparing siblings before other ceremonies and rituals that may be held around the baby's death can also be helpful, and parents may need assistance with this preparation.

Some funeral homes provide preparation and support for children. Britch (1996) reported on the Children's Room concept, which provides children with information on the grieving process, and Nilsen (2000) described the STAR Class as a way to prepare children for what will occur during the visitation or funeral service. If this type of service is not provided, families can prepare siblings similar to the way they were prepared to visit the NICU. The sensory approach provides siblings with information on what they will see and hear during the service, and the time-line approach provides them with information about what will happen first, second, third, and so on. Siblings can also benefit from a combination of these two approaches as well as having positive role models. As with any type of preparation, it is also important to consider the siblings' developmental level.

Providing Opportunities for Siblings to Participate

Siblings may want to assist family members as they prepare for the baby's funeral or memorial service, and there are several ways to involve them. For example, they might choose a special outfit for the baby to wear or a blanket to wrap around the baby. They can also help select flowers, toys, and pictures as well as music or readings. Some siblings may want to create special artwork or write a letter or poem.

Siblings may also appreciate opportunities to participate during the service. Fristad, Cerel, Goldman, Weller, and Weller (2000–2001) reported that children mentioned participation in the ceremony and ritual as being beneficial. Some of the ways that they can participate include handing out programs, lighting a candle, or reading a special prayer, poem, or letter. Siblings can also participate after the service, for instance, by helping to pick out a special headstone or memorial stone or planting flowers at the baby's graveside. They can also help greet people who might come to their home after the service and thank those who brought food and helped support their family throughout their ordeal.

Supporting Siblings During Ceremonies and Rituals

Having a familiar support person available during the ceremony for each sibling can be beneficial. Giovanola (2005) reported that the support person can allow parents to grieve and participate in the service with fewer distractions from siblings. The American Academy of Pediatrics (2000) discussed that support people can also provide siblings with preparation and assistance during the service. In addition, they can help siblings leave the service as needed, all of which can contribute to parents' worrying less about siblings' needs during the service.

Depending on siblings' developmental level, families may want to consider bringing a few toys or quiet activities to occupy siblings during downtimes or when they need a break. Parents or another adult may need to find a place for siblings to play that is close to where the family is gathered but far enough away that family and friends do not step on or trip over their things. If other children will be at the service, families might consider bringing extra toys, as children playing with toys tend to attract other children, and this is not the best time to expect siblings to share politely. Some funeral homes have play or activity rooms for children, complete with games, activities, and videos; however, it is important that siblings and other children do not feel they have been banished to these areas or to a play area set up by the family. Although children often need to take breaks from their grief, they continue to need their family's love and support during this time.

Supporting Siblings After Ceremonies and Rituals

Following the ceremonies and rituals, a large number of people may bring food and gather at the family's home to help support them. Mahon and Page (1995) mentioned that a few siblings described this as overwhelming or frightening. Young siblings may feel that people they do not know or people they do not know well are invading their home. It can also be difficult for siblings if extended family members or friends will be staying at their home, as this may cause their home routine to change even more than it already has. It can be especially difficult for siblings if they are required to share their room, bed, or toys during this stressful time.

Alternatives to Siblings
Attending the Funeral or Memorial Service

Although many professionals recommend giving siblings a choice about attending the funeral and other ceremonies and rituals, some parents may not be comfortable allowing their children to attend. Monroe and Kraus (1996) reported that it is not helpful to make parents feel guilty or that their children will develop long-term problems if they do not include them in these services. If parents are extremely uncomfortable with siblings attending these ceremonies and rituals, siblings will often be able to recognize their discomfort. These families may need suggestions for alternatives, such as having siblings say a private good-bye to the baby with their family before or following the public service, or joining their family in visits to the baby's graveside. Wilson (2001) described regular family visits to the baby's graveside with opportunities for siblings to be involved.

Special Activities and Traditions to Remember the Baby

Families may want to plan special activities or establish traditions as a way to remember the baby. Family members should be encouraged to communicate with one another and try several options to find what works best for their family.

- Fill a memory box with items to help siblings remember the baby. Items might include pictures of the baby, footprints or handprints, a lock of hair, a diaper or pacifier, and toys or Mylar balloons from the baby's bedside, particularly those that siblings picked out especially for the baby. Baby soap, shampoo, lotion, and oil can bring back pleasant baby smells in the future but should be packed carefully so they do not leak on other items in the memory box.

- Plant a memorial garden or tree in memory of the baby, although this may be difficult for siblings to leave behind should the family ever move.

- Give a remembrance gift in honor or in memory of the baby. The family may wish to donate funds or items in the baby's name to an agency that helps families that have babies who have been hospitalized in the NICU or in a hospice, who have a diagnosis similar to the diagnosis of the family's baby, or who have died.

- Create special traditions to celebrate the baby's birthday or the anniversary of the baby's death, or incorporate the memory of the baby into familiar family traditions. Siblings may have ideas or suggestions for ways to adapt family traditions in the years following the baby's death.

CONCLUSION

As families begin to recognize that their baby may die or after they have made the decision to utilize hospice services, they may request information from the health care team on ways to support the baby's siblings through this experience. Parents may also ask for assistance on how to support siblings during the funeral and other ceremonies following the baby's death. Many families can benefit from information on these issues, as well as finding options for additional sibling support in their local community. Also, because parents may have difficulty absorbing information that was delivered verbally at the hospital or hospice, it can be helpful to provide them with written information to refer to as needed in the future.

13

The Baby with Special Needs

Big Brother and Sister Issues

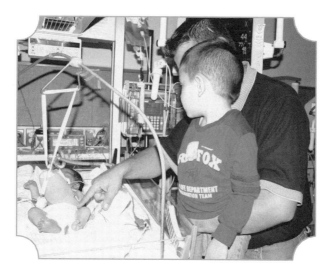

When a baby is discharged from the hospital with special needs, such as a disability or ongoing medical condition, and requires medical equipment at home, the entire family can be affected. Some issues can take time to integrate into the family's daily routines. Ray (2002) studied a small number of families with children who required at least one type of medical equipment. She reported that it took about 6 months for the child's medical and technical care to become a regular part of the family's routine and that the complexity of care did not appear to affect this time frame. Ray also stated that these families voiced concerns about the lack of time available to spend with siblings and that they attempted to find ways to spend quality time with all of their children.

POSITIVE INFLUENCES ON SIBLINGS

Having a child with special needs can be demanding and challenging, but it can also be a positive and growth-promoting experience for families (Dykens, 2005; McMillan, 2005; Stoneman, 2005). Hastings and Taunt (2002) reviewed research studies that discussed positive aspects of having a child with a disability in the family. They stated that even though these families can undergo more stress than families without children with disabilities, they can also have a variety of positive experiences. Miles, Holditch-Davis, Burchinal, and Nelson (1999) reported that mothers of high-risk babies experienced distress but also experienced growth.

Positive aspects for siblings of children with special needs have also begun to be explored. Meyer and Vadasy (1994) discussed that a child with a disability can influence siblings favorably, as well as contribute to their personal growth in a variety of areas, such as maturity, self-concept, tolerance, and advocacy. Pit-Ten Cate and Loots (2000) surveyed siblings of children with disabilities and reported that they had gained a more positive view of individuals who are different and of their parents as well. Fleitas (2000) discussed that siblings of children diagnosed with disabilities or an ongoing medical condition tend to be more mature, independent, and altruistic. According to Mandleco, Olsen, Dyches, and Marshall (2003), teachers of children who had siblings with disabilities rated them higher on issues such as self-control and cooperation than they rated children who did not have siblings with disabilities. If parents perceive the child with a disability in a positive light, siblings tend to view the child in a similar way (Strohm, 2005).

SIBLING DEVELOPMENTAL ISSUES

After the baby leaves the hospital and joins the family at home, parents may have significantly less time to spend with their other children. Siblings can therefore benefit from a continuation of the support and assistance they received during their mother's pregnancy and the baby's hospitalization. This can include maintaining familiar, consistent caregivers and regular routines, as well as providing developmentally appropriate explanations.

Older Infant and Toddler Siblings

Older infant and toddler siblings are learning many new skills such as cruising, walking, running, and climbing, as well as imitating their caregivers, as they explore their environment. If the baby requires medical equipment or supplies at home, safety issues should be considered. For example, the knobs, buttons, flashing lights, and beeping sounds on some medical equipment can be enticing to young siblings. If they observe their parents or other caregivers adjusting the buttons and knobs, they may decide to try it as well or may accidentally pull out cords or tubing. Families should be provided with information on safety options for the equipment, such as clear plastic covers. Smaller equipment and supplies should also be kept out of reach of siblings and the baby, and away from the edge of shelves or countertops where they can fall or be accidentally pulled off.

Older infant and toddler siblings and the baby are learning to build trusting relationships with their consistent caregivers. This can become more difficult if they are exposed to an increased number of inconsistent people, which can sometimes happen with a large home health team. Consistency in the members of the baby's home health care team can be beneficial whenever it is possible.

Preschool Siblings

Many preschool siblings are interested in the baby's medical equipment and can often benefit from a doll that has been adapted with medical equipment similar to the baby's. The doll can allow them to explore lines and tubing without endangering the baby. Preschool siblings of healthy, full-term babies often use dolls to imitate the way their parents feed, change, and care for the baby. Similarly, having a doll that is outfitted with medical equipment can provide preschool siblings of a baby with special needs with opportunities to more accurately imitate the way their parents care for the baby.

Preschool siblings also tend to notice when the baby attracts attention while out in public. Families may need assistance to help young siblings cope with this issue. Siblings will often use their parents and other family members as role models in these situations. Green (1996) reported that

Tip for Families

Develop a rehearsed statement your family shares with strangers when out in public. Make it simple enough or adapt it so that siblings can use it as well.

when families receive inappropriate comments or stares, the most important message is that which is given to the child with a disability, not the individual who stared or made the comment. The message and support that is given to siblings is just as important.

School-Age Siblings

School-age siblings are often beginning to have more experiences with peers, usually through school and organized activities. They can need support and assistance in sharing information about the baby's diagnosis or medical equipment with their friends, as well as coping with any of their friends' possibly insensitive remarks. Their friends may have limited or no experience with individuals who have special needs and may be unsure of how to react or respond. These siblings can also benefit from a doll adapted with the baby's medical equipment, not only as a way to help them better understand the equipment and the baby's situation, but also as a way to help them explain these issues to their friends. Some siblings might even be interested in assisting with these adaptations.

School-age siblings may also need support and assistance to cope with staring or inconsiderate remarks from strangers when their family is out in public with the baby.

Marina, age 6, was at the playground with her mother and her baby brother, who had a nasogastric tube. As her baby brother sat in his stroller near their mother, a large number of the children and adults who walked by stared at him, and some even walked by a second time for a better look or to ask questions. Marina responded by staying on the other side of the playground and pretending she did not know her brother. When it was time to leave, she walked several steps behind her mother and brother all the way home.

Eight-year-old Timothy left for the ice-cream shop with his father and baby sister with Down syndrome. While they were there, the family received second looks and several comments from some of the customers. On the way home, Timothy informed his father that he did not want to go get ice cream anymore if the baby went, too.

Nailah was at her soccer game with her mother and her baby sister, who required supplemental oxygen. Several members of the other team asked her questions about what was wrong with her sister. She repeated the answer that she and her parents had practiced: "My sister was born early and her lungs need some extra time to grow."

How families decide to handle these situations can vary according to parents' comfort levels, the family's cultural background, and the baby's diagnosis. Parents can often need assistance to view these situations from the sibling's perspective, as these occurrences can be more difficult for some siblings than for others.

Babies with special needs who have been discharged from the NICU often require regular follow-up appointments with a primary pediatrician. Occasionally, the siblings' current pediatrician is unable or unwilling to accept the baby's medical care, so the family is required to look for a new pediatrician. Some school-age siblings may want to be included in decisions regarding a new pediatrician, as some may have a history with their current pediatrician or feel that this may be just one more change they have to make because of the baby. For others, this change may not make a difference to them at all.

Preteen and Adolescent Siblings

Friends are important to many preteen and adolescent siblings, as is conforming with peer groups. Preteen and adolescent siblings may be uncomfortable when the baby attracts their friends' attention and may not know how to cope with friends' reactions. Some of their friends may be unsure of how to respond to a baby with special needs, whereas others may be excited about the new addition to the sibling's family. Some siblings may decide not to share information about the baby and related issues at home as a way of maintaining relationships that do not include the baby. Others may need assistance and support regarding ways to communicate information about the baby to their friends.

As with school-age siblings, preteen and adolescent siblings should be consulted if their primary pediatrician is unable or unwilling to accept the baby's care following discharge and the family is considering a new pediatrician. If siblings have a positive history with their current physician, they may not want to switch to a new one, although some siblings in this age group may be interested in switching to a physician who specializes in adolescents.

Many preteen and adolescent siblings are beginning to think about and imagine aspects of their future. Having a sibling with special needs may influence some of the choices they will make. Some siblings may feel that they should stay close to home to assist their family with caregiving issues rather than pursue higher education. In some families, the cost of the baby's medical and therapeutic expenses may also influence siblings' decisions regarding higher education. McHugh (2003), Meyer and Vadasy (1994), and Strohm (2005) discussed that having a child with special needs in the family can influence siblings' choices in occupations, where they will live, their marriage partners, and whether they will have children. These authors went on to say that many siblings choose occupations that assist and support people with disabilities and can often bring a unique perspective. Of a small number of siblings questioned by Baumann, Dyches, and Braddick (2005), those who mentioned future career plans listed helping occupations or going into business with their sibling with special needs.

EXTENDED FAMILY AND COMMUNITY SUPPORT SYSTEMS

The care of a baby with special needs following discharge is often a transition process for the entire family and can be more time consuming than many families anticipate. Parents are not only responsible for the baby's care, but also continue to be responsible for siblings' needs as well as household and job responsibilities. Dokken and Syndor-Greenberg (1998) discussed that families may need support as they incorporate the baby's care into an already busy family routine. They also mentioned that parents can become exhausted and overwhelmed and may require help to identify sources of support and assistance within the community.

In some cases, extended family members such as grandparents may join the household for a while to assist with a variety of duties. Grandparents of children with disabilities can also provide support in ways that can help strengthen family bonds. In addition, this can be a wonderful opportunity for siblings to spend quality time with a grandparent. Katz and Kessel (2002) questioned a small sample of grandparents whose grandchildren had developmental disabilities and reported that grandparents contributed many types of support and assistance, although the grandchildren's parents determined the amount of their involvement.

HOME HEALTH CARE

Home health care may be a new concept for many families at discharge, so they may have a variety of question and concerns when home health care issues are discussed. Families can often benefit from information about what has and has not been helpful for other families that have recently utilized home health care services. Although this information may give them ideas that may not have occurred to them otherwise, every family and situation is unique, and suggestions may be more beneficial for some families than for others.

One issue that is often different between the hospital and the home is the matter of boundaries. Home health care professionals share the caregiving role with the family to a much greater extent, as well as travel to the family's home and provide care on the family's turf. Corbett (1998) reported that in the hospital, parents are the visitors, whereas in the home, the professional assumes this role. In the home, families may notice a change in boundary issues, such as different opinions between the family and the home health care team on a variety of matters, including siblings' interactions with the baby as well as the role siblings will have in caring for the baby.

Murphy (1997) discussed that boundaries are an issue that many parents identify as a problem and that is often not addressed in discharge teaching. Kirk (2001) interviewed a small number of parents in the United Kingdom and reported that they had developed greater confidence in their ability to negotiate boundary issues with home health care professionals as time progressed and they gained more experience.

Cultural issues are also important. Beutter and Davidhizar (1999) and McNeil (1998) discussed that when home health care staff are unable to proficiently speak the family's language or the dialect of their language, communication problems can occur. It may not be as easy to obtain a translator in the home as it was in the hospital, and if siblings are expected to take on this role, it can deprive them of time socializing with peers or engaging in extracurricular activities at school. Beutter and Davidhizar and McNeil also discussed other cultural issues such as body language, communication styles, concept of time, beliefs about illness, folk medicine, religion, and the concept of family, all of which can influence the dynamics of home health care.

Siblings and Home Health Care Staff

Siblings need clear, concise, and developmentally appropriate explanations about the reasons for home health care. For very young siblings who may perceive that their home is being overrun or invaded by strangers, it can be beneficial to introduce them to members of the home health care team and include them in aspects of home health care. Older siblings may perceive experiences from the viewpoint of others. Baumgardner and Burtea (1998) organized focus groups of health care staff and members of families with children who used medical technology. A small number of older siblings and one adult sibling made up one of these groups and reported that it did not take them long to become accustomed to having the health care staff in their homes, and some siblings mentioned that they were able to recognize the support the staff provided their parents.

Members of the home health care staff may also become a significant source of support for families on a variety of sibling issues. They can develop trusting relationships with siblings and help them cope with the addition of the baby to the home environment. They can also assist families with safety issues, help siblings learn changes in the baby's medical care, promote positive interactions between siblings and the baby, and encourage individual time for parents and siblings.

Beginning and End of Home Health Care

Murphy (1997) discussed some of the phases families of high-risk infants can go through as they adjust to home health care following discharge. She reported that the first month appeared to be the most difficult and that it was not until after the first 6 months that families began to feel an increase in their comfort and confidence levels. This was due to some of the challenges that families had successfully dealt with during this time. Six months can be a long time for young siblings to wait for family life to become less stressful, especially when this time follows the baby's extended hospitalization. Murphy added that at 2 years following discharge, families often began to have difficulties with home health care issues again as they began to recognize that their child would need home health care support for an extended period.

The end of home health care can also be a difficult transition for many families. Agazio (1997) interviewed a small number of parents of children who used medical technology and had received at least 8 hours per week of home health care services for 3 months. These parents commented on the variety of emotions they experienced after they had gone through the transition of ending home health care services. They also discussed some of the issues that affected siblings when home health care services ended, including a reduction in the amount of time parents had to spend with siblings, loss of interaction with the home health care staff, and changes in routines.

When home health care services end, families will no longer see members of the staff on a regular basis, and siblings may want an opportunity to say good-bye. Families can often benefit from information on siblings' reactions to the end of home health care in advance to enable them to make arrangements to support siblings during this time. Arrangements might include providing familiar, consistent caregivers who can spend individual time with siblings or adapting family routines early so that changes can happen gradually and siblings can be involved in the process. It may also be helpful to provide opportunities for siblings to be involved in additional activities of their own, such as sports, scouts, art or dance classes, or extracurricular activities at school. If they are involved in these activities with a friend, their friend's family may be willing to provide or assist with transportation if this is a problem for the family.

FOLLOW-UP APPOINTMENTS AND EMERGENCY ISSUES

Babies with special needs and babies who use medical equipment at home can require numerous follow-up appointments after leaving the hospital. The frequency of these appointments can vary according to the baby's diagnosis and progress following discharge. Siblings may need to be prepared for the number of and reasons for these follow-up appointments to avoid possible misconceptions and misunderstandings. See Follow-Up Appointments in Chapter 11 for more information.

Families also need to anticipate emergency situations with the baby. One important issue is to identify caregivers who can be available to care for and support siblings at a moment's notice. Another issue might be the siblings' role in an emergency situation, which will greatly depend on siblings' age, maturity, coping skills, and available support systems. See Emergency Issues in Chapter 11 for more information.

REHOSPITALIZATION

Babies with special needs and babies who use medical technology at home can be at risk for rehospitalization depending on the baby's diagnosis and medical course. Rehospitalization may not always take place back in the NICU, where families are familiar with unit routines and have developed relationships with the staff. It may be possible to identify where in the hospital the baby may be readmitted before the initial discharge, which can allow parents and siblings to visit and learn about the new unit, as well as meet some of the staff. Becoming familiar with the new staff can also assist families as they support siblings and the baby during transitions from the home to the hospital environment and back. Information about the baby's rehospitalization during the discharge process, however, may be too overwhelming for some families. Their perception of rehospitalization at that point may be one of having failed to adequately care for their baby at home, so they may dismiss rehospitalization as a possibility.

During rehospitalizations, some families may want to continue to provide care for their baby, whereas others may want to use this time as a break from their caregiving responsibilities and spend it with siblings and as a couple. Some parents may want to divide the time between caring for the baby and being with siblings and each other. Parents should be encouraged to communicate the plans they believe best meet their family's needs.

If the baby requires readmission frequently or on a regular basis, it can become a regular part of the family's routine and parents may not notice its effects on siblings' coping and their need for information. Siblings' need for developmentally appropriate information and support can increase during these times, especially during critical aspects of the baby's hospitalizations. Some parents may believe that siblings already have an accurate and complete understanding of the baby's condition, and, therefore, communicating information may not be a high priority. Also, it can often be difficult for parents to assist siblings with their information needs when they may be coping with deteriorations in the baby's condition.

Additional support for siblings during this time includes the utilization of familiar, consistent caregivers and continuation of familiar family routines. Some babies may have to be rehospitalized without much notice, so families should consider providing caregivers for siblings and should identify them in advance, as parents and siblings can feel more comfortable when a tentative plan is in place. It can also be beneficial to discuss the baby's rehospitalization with siblings' teachers, who can also be a support system for siblings during this time.

RESPITE CARE

While the baby is still in the hospital, families may be too preoccupied to think about the assistance they can receive from a respite agency in the future. MacDonald and Callery (2004) stated that families reported that the respite care they received from family and friends began to decrease and that they had difficulty reciprocating the care as their child grew older. MacDonald and Callery also interviewed a small number of parents in the United Kingdom and reported that many of them benefited from respite care. Parents mentioned that it provided opportunities for them to spend time with siblings, spend time as a couple, catch up on their sleep, and rest, as well as have time as a regular family. Information on respite care can provide families with options for the future that can benefit both parents and siblings.

Different agencies can offer different types of respite care, and families should be encouraged to evaluate these services. Kendle and Campanale (2001) discussed a pediatric respite service that was coordinated in conjunction with a large church associated with a university and a school of nursing. They utilized nursing students who were able to provide consistent respite care for families throughout the semester, although there were certain skills they were unable to perform, such as dispensing medication. Also, the students could provide services only for children with special needs and not for siblings, but this enabled parents to spend additional time with siblings.

Appropriate respite care can be difficult for some families to locate or may be far from the family's home. Also, some services can have long waiting lists, and it may be months or even years before the family moves to the top of the list. Families should be encouraged to begin this process before respite care is desperately needed and parents are exhausted.

CONCLUSION

The support and information requirements siblings can have when a baby brother or sister with special needs is discharged home from the hospital tend to vary according to their developmental level. Other areas that can affect these issues include the baby's need for home health care, frequent follow-up appointments, and rehospitalizations. Families can often utilize the help of extended family members such as grandparents, community resources, and formal respite programs to provide needed assistance and support. The addition of a baby with special needs to the family can be a challenging experience, but it can be a positive growth experience as well.

Growing Together

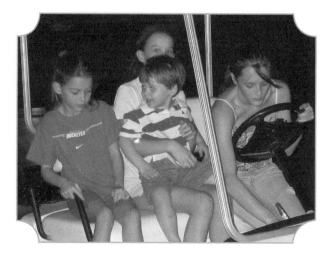

While the baby is hospitalized, siblings are often provided with information about the baby's condition, but their information needs tend to change as they grow and develop. For example, siblings who were toddlers when the baby was hospitalized will have different questions, concerns, and information needs about the baby's issues when they reach school age. Siblings may also revisit aspects of certain events in an attempt to gain a new understanding of them. Siblings' questions, concerns, and information needs can also be affected by changes in the baby's condition and development. Siblings can often benefit from opportunities to discuss not only the baby's hospital experience and past medical issues but also the baby's current medical issues.

Nathanial was 3 years old when his baby sister was born at 27 weeks gestation and spent several months in the NICU. At the time, Nathanial mainly asked questions about the baby's bed and toys. Now, at 11 years old, Nathanial is a sixth-grade student studying the different systems of the body in science class. When he began studying the reproductive system, he started to ask his parents questions about his sister's birth and NICU hospitalization.

Jessica was a toddler when her baby sister was born and hospitalized in the NICU with meconium aspiration syndrome. She is now 8 years old, and her best friend will soon be a new big sister. Jessica has been helping her best friend and her family as they prepare the nursery for their new baby. She has also begun to ask her parents a variety of questions about what happened when her sister was born.

Angel was 5 years old when his baby brother Luis was born and hospitalized in the NICU with severe respiratory distress syndrome. Luis spent some time on a ventilator before he was weaned to a nasal cannula and finally discharged home. Luis progressed very well at home until he was a toddler. One day, he had difficulty breathing, and his parents rushed him to the emergency center, where he went into respiratory distress. He was admitted to the pediatric intensive care unit and placed on a ventilator. Angel, at 7½ years old, began to compare Luis's current hospitalization with his initial hospitalization. He also asked his parents how he could be involved in Luis's care.

SIBLINGS' CONCERNS ABOUT THE FUTURE

Care needs for some babies may continue for long periods, and for those diagnosed with a disability, these needs may go on for the rest of their lives. As siblings mature, they can respond to this issue in different ways. Some may have the role of caregiver for an extended time, which may or may not be voluntary. Others may have limited involvement in the baby's care but continue to have a wonderful sibling relationship with the baby. Still others may have varying amounts of involvement in the baby's care over time due to changes in the siblings' and the baby's lives.

As siblings grow and develop, especially as they move into young adulthood, their knowledge and awareness of hereditary and genetic issues will likely increase, and they may begin to have additional questions and concerns, such as how their sibling's condition might affect their own children. Meyer and Vadasy (1994) discussed that as siblings grow older, they may become concerned that their own children could be born with or develop the same or similar problems as their sibling with disabilities. According to McHugh (2003), some siblings may feel comfortable about and capable of caring for a child of their own with special needs, whereas others may prefer not going through another experience with a child with special needs, and still others may be somewhere in between. Strohm (2005) reported that siblings may have concerns not only about their own children possibly having special needs, but also about their ability to care for their own children in addition to their sibling with disabilities when their parents no longer can. McHugh, Meyer and Vadasy, and Strohm also mentioned that siblings' experience with a child with special needs can influence their future relationships and career choices as well.

Siblings may also have concerns about pregnancy and childbearing issues. Those who have observed their mother's high-risk or difficult pregnancies may wonder about their own or their significant other's pregnancies, as well as health risks for children of such pregnancies. These siblings may want to look into genetic and prenatal counseling long before they consider having children.

Some babies who were hospitalized in the NICU may be rehospitalized repeatedly as they move into childhood. Doyle, Ford, and Davis (2003); Leijon, Finnstrom, Sydsjo, and Wadsby (2003); and Petrou et al. (2003) reported that preterm babies were readmitted to the hospital more often than full-term babies over the first few years of life. As the baby matures, siblings should continue to be supported and prepared for possible rehospitalizations and provided with information and opportunities to be involved. Many children's hospitals have child life specialists available who can assist families with these issues.

GENERAL SIBLING DEVELOPMENTAL ISSUES

After families have adjusted to the baby being home, they may need assistance balancing siblings' developmental needs with the baby's various care needs. The baby's needs are often the most important concern for families upon the baby's discharge, and for some, this may continue to be the case for months or even years. These families may require support and assistance meeting the needs of all family members. For example, siblings need opportunities to participate in developmentally appropriate activities, as well as to have interests apart from the baby and their role as a big brother or sister. Busy families may have to be reminded to acknowledge siblings' activities and interests and to celebrate their successes, accomplishments, struggles, and efforts and not let their issues be overshadowed by the baby's. Families should also be encouraged to continue to provide opportunities for siblings and the growing baby to interact in a positive way to help build and strengthen their relationship in the years to come.

FAMILY ISSUES

Siblings' coping abilities change as they mature and their life experiences multiply. They can benefit from continued assistance and support in developing effective coping skills to deal with stressful situations, whether they are related to the baby's or their own experiences. The baby's coping skills will also develop and change and often be quite different from their older siblings' coping style, which can be challenging for parents.

Families should be encouraged to maintain an environment of honest and open communication in which siblings can feel safe and comfortable asking questions, requesting information, and expressing their emotions. Siblings may also need assistance and support explaining some of the baby's issues, such as rehospitalization, developmental delays, or disabilities, with their friends and classmates. Teachers in coming years may also need to be informed if the baby has long-term issues. Also, as siblings get older, they may often want a voice in deciding what information is shared with their teachers and classmates.

Various family and child safety issues should be addressed periodically as siblings and the baby grow and develop or as the baby's condition changes. Family interactions will continue to change, as well as family interests and activities. When safety issues should be introduced can vary with siblings' and the baby's developmental levels and experiences. Parents may need information on safety issues not only in their home but in other environments as well.

MOVING PAST THE NICU EXPERIENCE

Many families take pictures or videos during the baby's hospitalization as a way to remember the experience or to share with family and friends. Wilson, Munson, Koel, and Hitterdahl (1987) looked at families' responses when mothers shared these photographs with their children who had been hospitalized as babies in the NICU and were now between the ages of 3 and 7. The mothers reported that their children had numerous questions about the photographs regarding the medical equipment, their size and coloration as babies, whether they were in pain, if they were left alone, and so forth. When siblings and the child who was in the hospital begin to ask additional questions about NICU experience, these photographs can allow parents to share information visually about different aspects of it. In addition, photographs taken in the hospital, along with family photographs taken on a periodic or regular basis, can help families see how far they have come and some of the changes that have occurred since the baby's hospitalization, as well as provide a time line of the baby's growth and development.

CONCLUSION

After they have adapted to the baby being home, family members should be encouraged to continue with family life and begin to make new family memories. It is important to include the baby in family activities, routines, and rituals on a regular basis, even if they have to be adapted to accommodate the baby's needs. As the sibling and baby continue to grow and develop, these routines, rituals, and activities can help provide memories that include the entire family and that can become special to each family member.

References

Agazio, J.G. (1997). Family transition through the termination of private duty home care nursing. *Journal of Pediatric Nursing, 12,* 74–84.

Ahmann, E. (1997). Books for siblings of children having illness or disability. *Pediatric Nursing, 23,* 500–502.

Ahmann, E. (2000). Supporting families' savvy use of the Internet for health research. *Pediatric Nursing, 26,* 419–423.

American Academy of Child and Adolescent Psychiatry. (2005a). *Children and grief.* Retrieved October 12, 2005, from http://www.aacap.org/publications/factsfam/grief.htm

American Academy of Child and Adolescent Psychiatry. (2005b). *Knowing when to seek help for your child.* Retrieved October 12, 2005, from http://www.aacap.org/publications/factsfam/whenhelp.htm

American Academy of Pediatrics. (1985). Committee on fetus and newborn: Postpartum (neonatal) sibling visitation. *Pediatrics, 76,* 650.

American Academy of Pediatrics. (1998). Hospital discharge of the high-risk neonate—proposed guidelines [Electronic version]. *Pediatrics, 102,* 411–417.

American Academy of Pediatrics. (2000). The pediatrician and childhood bereavement [Electronic version]. *Pediatrics, 105,* 445–447.

American Academy of Pediatrics. (n.d.). *Mat release, toy safety: Put these tips on your list.* Retrieved August 21, 2005, from http://www.aap.org/pressroom/toymatrelease.pdf

American Society for Reproductive Medicine. (2003). *Patient's fact sheet: Challenges of parenting multiples.* Retrieved October 12, 2005, from http://www.asrm.org/Patients/FactSheets/challenges.pdf

Anderberg, G.J. (1988). Initial acquaintance and attachment behavior of siblings with the newborn. *Journal of Obstetric, Gynecologic, and Neonatal Nursing, 17,* 49–54.

Andrade, T.M. (1998). Sibling visitation: Research implications for pediatric and neonatal patients [Electronic version]. *Online Journal of Knowledge Synthesis for Nursing, 5,* 58–64.

Ayyash-Abdo, H. (2001). Childhood bereavement: What school psychologists need to know. *School Psychology International, 22,* 417–433.

Baer, N.A. (1996). Cardiopulmonary resuscitation on television: Exaggerations and accusations. *New England Journal of Medicine, 334,* 1604–1605.

Ballard, J.L., Maloney, M., Shank, M., & Hollister, L. (1984). Sibling visits to a newborn intensive care unit: Implications for siblings, parents, and infants. *Child Psychiatry and Human Development, 14,* 203–214.

Barrett, A., & Schuurman, D.L. (2000). The power of choice: Understanding the needs of children in funeral planning and services. *The Director, 72,* 50–53.

Baumann, S.L., Dyches, T.T., & Braddick, M. (2005). Being a sibling. *Nursing Science Quarterly, 18,* 51–58.

Baumgardner, D.J., & Burtea, E.D. (1998). Quality-of-life in technology-dependent children receiving home care, and their families—a qualitative study. *Wisconsin Medical Journal, 97,* 51–55.

Berns, C.F. (2004). Bibliotherapy: Using books to help bereaved children. *Omega: Journal of Death and Dying, 48,* 321–336.

Beutter, M.B., & Davidhizar, R. (1999). A home care provider's challenge—caring for the Hispanic client in the home. *Journal of Practical Nursing, 49,* 26–33.

Blondel, B., & Kaminski, M. (2002). Trends in the occurrence, determinants, and consequences of multiple births. *Seminars in Perinatology, 26,* 239–249.

Brazy, J.E., Anderson, B.M.H., Becker, P.T., & Becker, M. (2001). How parents of premature infants gather information and obtain support. *Neonatal Network, 20,* 41–48.

Britch, C. (1996). The children's room. *The Director, 68,* 28–30.

Brooks, B.A. (2001). Using the Internet for patient education. *Orthopaedic Nursing, 20,* 69–77.

Bryan, E. (2003). The impact of multiple preterm births on the family. *Hospital Medicine, 64,* 648–650.

Busch, T., & Kimble, C.S. (2001). Grieving children: Are we meeting the challenge? *Pediatric Nursing, 27,* 414–418.

Campbell, D., van Teijlingen, E.R., & Yip, L. (2004). Economic and social implications of multiple birth. *Best Practice & Research Clinical Obstetrics and Gynaecology, 18,* 657–668.

Carbonell-Estrany, X., Quero, J., Bustos, G., Cotero, A., Domenech, E., Figueras-Aloy, J., et al. (2000). Rehospitalization because of respiratory syncytial virus infection in premature infants younger than 33 weeks of gestation: A prospective study. *Pediatric Infections Disease Journal, 19,* 592–597.

Christ, G.H. (2000). Impact of development on children's mourning. *Cancer Practice, 8,* 72–81.

Cohen, L.J. (1987). Bibliotherapy using literature to help children deal with difficult problems. *Journal of Psychosocial Nursing and Mental Health Services, 25,* 20–24.

Compassionate Friends. (2003, October 14). *When a child in your school is bereaved.* Retrieved March 2, 2005, from http://www.tcf.org.uk/leaflets/leschools.html

Corbett, N.A. (1998). Homecare, technology, and the management of respiratory disease. *Critical Care Nursing Clinics of North America, 10,* 305–313.

Davies, L. (2003). *Using bibliotherapy with children.* Retrieved February 10, 2006, from http://www.kellybear.com/TeacherArticles/TeacherTip34.html

Deering, C.G., & Cody, D.J. (2002). Communication with children and adolescents. *American Journal of Nursing, 102,* 34–41.

DeMaso, D.R., Meyer, E.C., & Beasley, P.J. (1997). What do I say to my surviving children? *Journal of the American Academy of Child Adolescent Psychiatry, 36,* 1299–1302.

Dhillon, A.S., Albersheim, S.G., Alsaad, S., Pargass, N.S., & Zupancic, J.A.F. (2003). Internet use and perceptions of information reliability by parents in a neonatal intensive care unit. *Journal of Perinatology, 23,* 420–424.

Diem, S.J., Lantos, J.D., & Tulsky, J.A. (1996). Cardiopulmonary resuscitation on television miracles and misinformation. *New England Journal of Medicine, 334,* 1578–1582.

Dokken, D.L., & Sydnor-Greenberg, N. (1998). Helping families mobilize their personal resources. *Pediatric Nursing, 24,* 66–69.

Dougy Center for Grieving Children, The. (2003). *Helping the grieving student: A guide for teachers.* Portland, OR: Author.

Doyle, L.W., Ford, G., & Davis, N. (2003). Health and hospitalizations after discharge in extremely low birth weight infants. *Seminars in Neonatology, 8,* 137–145.

Drake, E. (1999). Internet technology: Resources for perinatal nurses. *Journal of Obstetric, Gynecologic, and Neonatal Nursing, 28,* 15–21.

Dykens, E.M. (2005). Happiness, well-being, and character strengths: Outcomes for families and siblings of persons with mental retardation. *Mental Retardation, 43,* 360–364.

Elder, D.E., Hagan, R., Evans, S.F., Benninger, H.R., & French, N.P. (1999). Hospital admissions in the first year of life in very preterm infants. *Journal of Paediatrics and Child Health, 35,* 145–150.

Escobar, G.J., Greene, J.D., Hulac, P., Kincannon, E., Bischoff, K., Gardner, M.N., et al. (2005). Rehospitalization after birth hospitalization: Patterns among infants of all gestations. *Archives of Disease in Childhood, 90,* 125–131.

Escobar, G.J., Joffe, S., Gardner, M.N., Armstrong, M.A., Folck, B.F., & Carpenter, D.M. (1999). Rehospitalization in the first two weeks after discharge from the neonatal intensive care unit [Electronic version]. *Pediatrics, 104,* e2.

Espeland, K. (1998). Promoting mental wellness in children and adolescents through positive coping mechanisms. *Journal of School Nursing, 14,* 22–25.

Fiese, B.H. (2002). Routines of daily living and rituals in family life: A glimpse at stability and changes during the early child-raising years. *Zero to Three, 22,* 10–13.

Fleitas, J. (2000). When Jack fell down… Jill came tumbling after: Siblings in the web of illness and disability. *American Journal of Maternal/Child Nursing, 25,* 267–273.

Foley, M. (1996a). *Older siblings of multiples.* Retrieved February 25, 2005, from http://www.twinslist.org/sibling.htm

Foley, M. (1996b). *Older siblings of multiples continued…* Retrieved February 25, 2005, from http://www.twinslist.org/sibling2.htm

Free, C., Green, J., Bhavnani, V., & Newman, A. (2003). Bilingual young people's experiences of interpreting in primary care: A qualitative study. *British Journal of General Practice, 53,* 530–535.

Fristad, M.A., Cerel, J., Goldman, M., Weller, E.B., & Weller, R.A. (2000–2001). The role of ritual in children's bereavement. *Omega: Journal of Death and Dying, 42,* 321–339.

Fry, M.J., Cartwright, D.W., Huang, R.C., & Davies, M.W. (2003). Preterm birth: A long distance from home and its significant social and financial stress. *Australian and New Zealand Journal of Obstetrics and Gynaecology, 43,* 317–321.

Gavin, M.L. (Reviewer). (2004, November). *Teaching your child how to use 911.* Retrieved June 28, 2005, from http://kidshealth.org/parent/positive/family/911.html

Giovanola, J. (2005). Sibling involvement at the end of life. *Association of Pediatric Oncology Nurses, 22,* 222–236.

Gordon, P.N., Williamson, S., & Lawler, P.G. (1998). As seen on TV: Observational study of cardiopulmonary resuscitation in British television medical dramas [Electronic version]. *British Medical Journal, 317,* 780–783.

Green, J. (1996). *This one is about: Reaction time.* Retrieved June 19, 2005, from http://www.widesmiles.org/outreach/ws009.html

Green, J., Free, C., Bhavnani, V., & Newman, T. (2005). Translators and mediators: Bilingual young people's accounts of their interpreting work in health care. *Social Science & Medicine, 60,* 2097–2110.

Griffin, T., Kavanaugh, K., Soto, C.F., & White, M. (1997). Parental evaluation of a tour of the neonatal intensive care unit during a high-risk pregnancy [Electronic version]. *Journal of Obstetric, Gynecologic, and Neonatal Nursing, 26,* 59–65.

Haddon, L.P. (2000). *The singleton siblings of multiples.* Retrieved February 25, 2005, from http://www.multiplebirthsfamilies.com/articles/post_q3.html

Hames, C.C. (2003). Helping infants and toddlers when a family member dies [Electronic version]. *Journal of Hospice and Palliative Nursing, 5,* 103–110.

Hamrick, W.B., & Reilly, L. (1992). A comparison of infection rates in a newborn intensive care unit before and after adoption of open visitation. *Neonatal Network, 11,* 15–18.

Hansdottir, I., & Malcarne, V.L. (1998). Concepts of illness in Icelandic children. *Journal of Pediatric Psychology, 23,* 187–195.

Hastings, R.P., & Taunt, H.M. (2002). Positive perceptions in families of children with developmental disabilities. *American Journal on Mental Retardation, 107,* 116–127.

Holland, J. (2004). Should children attend their parent's funerals? *Pastoral Care in Education, 22,* 10–14.

Jensen, V.K. (1995). Children's conceptualization of illness: Translating data into practice. *Clinical Pediatrics, 34,* 183–184.

Johnson, A.H. (1997). Death in the PICU: Caring for the "other" families. *Journal of Pediatric Nursing, 12,* 273–277.

Katz, S., & Kessel, L. (2002). Grandparents of children with developmental disabilities: Perceptions, beliefs, and involvement in their care. *Issues in Comprehensive Pediatric Nursing, 25,* 113–128.

Kendle, J., & Campanale, R. (2001). A pediatric learning experience: Respite care for families with children with special needs. *Nurse Educator, 26,* 95–98.

Kirk, S. (2001). Negotiating lay and professional roles in the care of children with complex health care needs. *Journal of Advanced Nursing, 34,* 593–602.

Kollantai, J.A., & Fleischer, L.M. (1993). *Multiple birth loss and the hospital caregiver.* Retrieved October 12, 2005, from http://www.climb-support.org/pdf/mblnicu.pdf

Kowba, M.D., & Schwirian, P.M. (1985). Direct sibling contact and bacterial colonization in newborns. *Journal of Obstetric, Gynecologic, and Neonatal Nursing, 14,* 412–417.

Kramer, L. (1996). What's real in children's fantasy play? Fantasy play across the transition to becoming a sibling. *Journal of Child Psychology and Psychiatry, 37,* 329–337.

Kramer, L., & Schaefer-Hernan, P. (1994). Patterns of fantasy play engagement across the transition to becoming a sibling. *Journal of Child Psychology and Psychiatry, 35,* 749–767.

Lamarche-Vadel, A., Blondel, B., Truffert, P., Burguet, A., Cambonie, G., Selton, D., et al. (2004). Re-hospitalization in infants younger than 29 weeks' gestation in the EPIPAGE cohort. *Acta Paediatrica, 93,* 1340–1345.

Lamp, L.J., & Howard, P.A. (1999). Guiding parents' use of the Internet for newborn education. *American Journal of Maternal/Child Nursing, 24,* 33–36.

Laws, M.B., Heckscher, R., Mayo, S.J., Li, W., & Wilson, I.B. (2004). A new method for evaluating the quality of medical interpretation. *Medical Care, 42,* 71–80.

Leijon, I., Finnstrom, O., Sydsjo, G., & Wadsby, M. (2003). Use of healthcare resources, family function, and socioeconomic support during the first four years after preterm birth [Electronic version]. *Archives of Disease in Childhood: Fetal & Neonatal Edition, 88,* F415–F420.

Levine, C., Glajchen, M., & Cournos, F. (2004). A fifteen-year-old translator. *Hastings Center Report, 34,* 10–12.

Lobato, D.J., & Koa, B.T. (2002). Integrated sibling–parent group intervention to improve sibling knowledge and adjustment to chronic illness and disability. *Journal of Pediatric Psychology, 27,* 711–716.

Lobato, D.J., & Koa, B.T. (2005). Brief report: Family-based group intervention for young siblings of children with chronic illness and developmental disability. *Journal of Pediatric Psychology, 30,* 678–682.

MacDonald, H., & Callery, P. (2004). Different meanings of respite: A study of parents, nurses and social workers caring for children with complex needs. *Child: Care, Health & Development, 30,* 279–288.

MacWhinney, K., Cermak, S.A., & Fisher, A. (1987). Body part identification in 1- to 4-year-old children. *American Journal of Occupational Therapy, 41,* 454–459.

Mahon, M.M. (1994). Death of a sibling: Primary care interventions. *Pediatric Nursing, 20,* 293–295, 328.

Mahon, M.M., & Page, M.L. (1995). Childhood bereavement after the death of a sibling. *Holistic Nursing Practice, 9,* 15–26.

Maloni, J.A., Brezinski-Tomasi, J.E., & Johnson, L.A. (2001). Antepartum bed rest: Effect upon the family. *Journal of Obstetric, Gynecologic, and Neonatal Nursing, 30,* 165–173.

Maloni, J.A., & Kutil, R.M. (2000). Antepartum support group for women hospitalized on bed rest. *American Journal of Maternal/Child Nursing, 25,* 204–210.

Mandleco, B., Olsen, S.F., Dyches, T., & Marshall, E. (2003). The relationship between family and sibling functioning in families raising a child with a disability. *Journal of Family Nursing, 9,* 365–396.

Manworren, R.C.B., & Woodring, B. (1998). Evaluating children's literature as a source for patient education. *Pediatric Nursing, 24,* 548–553.

Mariano, C., & Hickey, R. (1998). Multiple pregnancy, multiple needs. *Canadian Nurse, 94,* 26–30.

Maroney, D.I. (1995). Realities of a premature infant's first year: Helping parents cope. *Journal of Perinatology, 15,* 418–422.

Martin, J.A., Hamilton, B.E., Sutton, P.D., Ventura, S.J., Menacker, F., & Munson, M.L. (2005). *Births: Final data for 2003. National Vital Statistics Reports 54.* Retrieved October 9, 2005, from www.cdc.gov/nchs/data/nvsr/nvsr54/nvsr54_02.pdf

May, K.A. (2001). Impact of prescribed activity restriction during pregnancy on women and families. *Health Care for Women International, 22,* 29–47.

McCartney, P.R. (2004). Sidelines—supporting mothers on bed rest. *American Journal of Maternal/Child Nursing, 29,* 405.

McHaffie, H.E., Lyon, A.J., & Fowlie, P.W. (2001). Lingering death after treatment withdrawal in the neonatal intensive care unit [Electronic version]. *Archives of Disease in Childhood: Fetal & Neonatal Edition, 85,* 8–12.

McHugh, M. (2003). *Special siblings: Growing up with someone with a disability* (Rev. ed.). Baltimore: Paul H. Brookes Publishing Co.

McMillan, E. (2005). A parent's perspective. *Mental Retardation, 43,* 351–353.

McNeil, G.J. (1998). Diversity issues in the homecare setting. *Critical Care Nursing Clinics of North America, 10,* 357–368.

Meyer, D.J., & Vadasy, P.F. (1994). *Sibshops: Workshops for siblings of children with special needs.* Baltimore: Paul H. Brookes Publishing Co.

Meyer, E.C., Kennally, K.F., Zika-Beres, E., Cashore, W.J., & Oh, W. (1996). Attitudes about sibling visitation in the neonatal intensive care unit. *Archives of Pediatric Adolescent Medicine, 150,* 1021–1026.

Miles, M.S., Holditch-Davis, D., Burchinal, P., & Nelson, D. (1999). Distress and growth outcomes in mothers of medically fragile infants. *Nursing Research, 48,* 129–140.

Minnesota Poison Control System. (2004). *Seniors and medication safety.* Retrieved July 18, 2005, from http://www.mnpoison.org/index.asp?pageID=207

Monroe, B., & Kraus, F. (1996). Children and loss. *British Journal of Hospital Medicine, 56,* 260–264.

Montgomery, L.A., Kleiber, C., Nicholson, A., & Craft-Rosenberg, M. (1997). A research-based sibling visitation program for the neonatal ICU. *Critical Care Nursing, 17,* 29–35, 38–40.

Munch, S., & Levick, J. (2001). "I'm special, too": Promoting sibling adjustment in the neonatal intensive care unit. *Health & Social Work, 26,* 58–64.

Murphy, K.E. (1997). Parenting a technology assisted infant: Coping with occupational stress. *Social Work in Health Care, 24,* 113–126.

Myant, K.A., & Williams, J.A. (2005). Children's concepts of health and illness: Understanding of contagious illnesses, non-contagious illnesses and injuries. *Journal of Health Psychology, 10,* 805–819.

Ngo-Metzger, Q., Massagil, M.P., Clarridge, B.R., Manocchia, M., Davis, R.B., Iezzoni, L.I., et al. (2003). Linguistic and cultural barriers to care perspectives of Chinese and Vietnamese immigrants. *Journal of General Internal Medicine, 18,* 44–52.

Nilsen, K.E. (2000). The STAR class. *The Director, 72,* 48–50.

Oehler, J.M., & Vileisis, R.A. (1990). Effect of early sibling visitation in an intensive care nursery. *Developmental and Behavior Pediatrics, 11,* 7–12.

Pector, E.A. (2004). Views of bereaved multiple-birth parents on live support decisions, the dying process, and discussions surrounding death. *Journal of Perinatology, 24,* 4–10.

Pector, E.A., & Smith-Levitin, M. (2002a, March). Bereavement in multiple birth. Part 1: General considerations [Electronic version]. *The Female Patient.* Retrieved October 12, 2005, from http://www.femalepatient.com/html/arc/sel/ march02/article02.asp

Pector, E.A., & Smith-Levitin, M. (2002b, April). Bereavement in multiple birth. Part 2: Dual dilemmas [Electronic version]. *The Female Patient.* Retrieved October 12, 2005, from http://www.femalepatient.com/html/arc/sel/april02/article05.asp

Peebles-Kleiger, M.J. (2000). Pediatric and neonatal intensive care hospitalization as traumatic stressor: Implications for intervention. *Bulletin of the Menninger Clinic, 64,* 257–280.

Petrou, S., Mehta, Z., Hockley, C., Cook-Mozaffari, P., Henderson, J., & Goldacre, M. (2003). The impact of preterm birth on hospital inpatient admissions and costs during the first 5 years of life [Electronic version]. *Pediatrics, 112,* 1290–1297.

Pettle, S.A., & Britten, C.M. (1995). Talking with children about death and dying. *Child: Care, Health and Development, 21,* 395–404.

Pit-Ten Cate, I.M., & Loots, G.M. (2000). Experiences of siblings of children with physical disabilities: An empirical investigation. *Disability and Rehabilitation, 22,* 399–408.

Raman, L., & Gelman, S.A. (2005). Children's understanding of the transmission of genetic disorders and contagious illnesses. *Developmental Psychology, 41,* 171–182.

Ray, L.D. (2002). Parenting and childhood chronicity: Making visible the invisible work. *Journal of Pediatric Nursing, 17,* 424–438.

Ritchie, S.K. (2002). Primary care of the premature infant discharged from the neonatal intensive care unit. *American Journal of Maternal/ChildNursing, 27,* 76–85.

Rozdilsky, J.R. (2005). Enhancing sibling presence in pediatric ICU. *Critical Care Nursing Clinics of North America, 17,* 451–461.

Rubel, B. (2005). Identifying ways school nurses can support grieving children and adolescents. *School Nurse News, 22,* 28–34.

Russell, R.B., Petrini, J.R., Damus, K., Mattison, D.R., & Schwarz, R.H. (2003). The changing epidemiology of multiple births in the United States. *Obstetrics & Gynecology, 101,* 129–135.

Santoro, M., & Bennett-Santoro, P. (n.d.). *For brothers and sisters talking to teachers about grief.* Retrieved March 10, 2005, from http://www.climb-support.org/pdf/talkingtoteachers.pdf

Sawicki, J.A. (1997). Sibling rivalry and the new baby: Anticipatory guidance and management strategies. *Pediatric Nursing, 23,* 298–302.

Schwab, F., Tolbert, B., Bagnato, S., & Maisels, M.J. (1983). Sibling visiting in a neonatal intensive care unit. *Pediatrics, 71,* 835–838.

Sibling Support Project, The. (n.d.). University of Washington survey: Positive results of Sibshops last into adulthood. Retrieved February 22, 2006, from http://www.thearc.org/siblingsupport/uwsurvey

Solheim, K., & Spellacy, C. (1988). Sibling visitation: Effects on newborn infection rates. *Journal of Obstetric, Gynecologic, and Neonatal Nursing, 17,* 43–48.

Stoneman, Z. (2005). Siblings of children with disabilities: Research themes. *Mental Retardation, 43,* 339–350.

Strohm, K. (2005). *Being the other one: Growing up with a brother or sister who has special needs.* Boston: Shambhala.

Stuber, M.L., & Mesrkhani, V.H. (2001). "What do we tell the children?" Understanding childhood grief [Electronic version]. *Western Journal of Medicine, 174,* 187–191.

Tichon, J., & Yellowless, P. (2003). Internet social support for children and adolescents. *Journal of Telemedicine and Telecare, 9,* 238–240.

Umphenour, J.H. (1980). Bacterial colonization in neonates with sibling visitation. *Journal of Obstetrics, Gynecologic, and Neonatal Nursing, 9,* 73–75.

U.S. Consumer Product Safety Commission. (n.d.). *CPSC warns consumers of suffocation danger associated with children's balloons.* Retrieved August 21, 2005, from http://www.cpsc.gov/cpscpub/pubs/5087.pdf

Van den Bulck, J.J. (2002). The impact of television fiction on public expectations of survival following in-hospital cardiopulmonary resuscitation by medical professionals. *European Journal of Emergency Medicine, 9,* 325–329.

Van den Bulck, J., & Damiaans, K. (2004). Cardiopulmonary resuscitation on Flemish television: Challenges to the television effects hypothesis [Electronic version]. *Emergency Medicine Journal, 21,* 565–567.

VandenBerg, K.A. (1999). What to tell parents about the developmental needs of their baby at discharge. *Neonatal Network, 18,* 57–59.

Verma, R.P., Sridhar, S., & Spitzer, A.R. (2003). Continuing care of NICU graduates. *Clinical Pediatrician, 42,* 299–315.

Volling, B.L. (2005). The transition to siblinghood: A developmental ecological systems perspective and directions for future research. *Journal of Family Psychology, 19,* 542–549.

Wallinga, C., & Skeen, P. (1996). Siblings of hospitalized and ill children: The teacher's role in helping these forgotten family members. *Young Children, 51,* 78–83.

Weaver, J. (1996). *Focus on siblings.* Retrieved October 6, 2005, from http://www.parentsinc.org/newsletter/Dec96/Focus.html

Williams, J.M., & Binnie, L.M. (2002). Children's concepts of illness: An intervention to improve knowledge. *British Journal of Health Psychology, 7,* 129–147.

Williams, R.L., & Medalie, J.H. (1994). Twins: Double pleasure or double trouble? *American Family Physician, 49,* 869–873.

Wilson, A.L., Munson, D.P., Koel, D., & Hitterdahl, M. (1987). Mothers and their children look at baby pictures: The NICU experience in retrospect. *Clinical Pediatrics, 26,* 576–580.

Wilson, R.E. (2001). Parents' support of their children after a miscarriage or perinatal death. *Early Human Development, 61,* 55–65.

Wranesh, B.L. (1982). The effect of sibling visitation on bacterial colonization rate in neonates. *Journal of Obstetric, Gynecologic, and Neonatal Nursing, 11,* 211–213.

Yantzi, N., Rosenberg, M.W., Burke, S.O., & Harrison, M.B. (2001). The impacts of distance to hospital on families with a child with a chronic condition. *Social Science & Medicine, 52,* 1777–1791.

Zeitlin, S.V. (2001). Grief and bereavement. *Primary Care: Clinics in Office Practice, 28,* 415–425.

Resources

SUGGESTIONS FOR WAYS TO
SUPPORT SIBLINGS AND THEIR FAMILIES

Some families may be inundated with offers of assistance and support when the mother is placed on bed rest, as well as following the baby's admission to the hospital, the discharge home, or, in some cases, the baby's death. Many families may be too overwhelmed to know where to start or what to suggest to those who offer assistance and support. Others may find that it is more difficult to communicate information and delegate tasks than it is to take care of matters themselves. Dokken and Sydnor-Greenberg (1998) suggested that families designate an individual to help them coordinate this assistance, although it may be difficult to find someone who can assume this role. Instead, families may want to consider creating a list of ways in which extended family members and family friends who are willing and able can assist and support them during this time. The following suggestions include ideas that families have used in the past and that families may want to include on their list.

Helping Siblings

- Provide fun activities with siblings on a regular or as-needed basis, which can give siblings special time with a caring, familiar, consistent adult when parents need a break or when they are unable to provide this kind of support.

- Send siblings special surprises in the mail on a regular or as-needed basis. Receiving a package in the mail can be a big deal for siblings and can help them feel remembered when the family's primary focus is the baby. Items should be able to fit in the family's mailbox so that a trip to the post office can be avoided.

- Assist siblings with schoolwork, such as homework, special projects, and studying for tests.

- Take the family's turn at driving in the car pool or provide transportation to extracurricular activities.

- Be the siblings' special cheering section at extracurricular activities, such as ball games, recitals, concerts, or presentations, especially if parents are unable to be there.

- Provide familiar, kid-friendly breakfast foods to help siblings get school mornings off to a good start, and supply special lunch items.

- Depending on siblings' desires, offer transportation to and from church, synagogue, mosque, or other religious institutions, especially when parents are unable to attend.

- Recognize siblings when acknowledging the baby's birth or death. A small bouquet of flowers, a cookie bouquet, a balloon, or a small gift addressed to siblings can help them feel special and remembered.

Helping Parents

- Assist with housecleaning, minor home repairs, laundry, yard work, car washing or repair, and pet care, as well as shopping for groceries and running errands. This can help increase the amount of time that parents can spend with siblings.

- Provide gift certificates to restaurants, especially those with kid-friendly food that deliver.

- Provide familiar, kid-friendly frozen dinners so that parents can easily put a meal on the table and have extra time to spend with siblings.

- Provide memberships to places that the family can enjoy together, such as museums, zoos, arts and crafts events, amusement parks, activity centers, or movies.

- Assist parents in maintaining daily family routines as well as family rituals, such as holiday and sibling birthday celebrations.

- Provide assistance and support on holidays, as home health care staff may not be available.

Helping with Medical Care

- Stay with siblings while parents learn the baby's care, as well as after the baby's discharge during follow-up appointments, rehospitalizations, and medical emergencies.

- Learn the baby's care to provide parents with opportunities to spend quality time with siblings and with each other. Do not be offended if it takes time before parents are comfortable accepting your offer.

- Provide rides to and from the hospital, or assist with the cost of gas, parking, or public transportation, as this expense can limit family visitations. Families can also benefit from similar assistance during follow-up visits after the baby's discharge.

- Throw a "coming home" shower with items for the baby and siblings. Babies who have been hospitalized may need special formulas and other items not covered by insurance. Siblings often feel special when they are remembered, too.

GUIDELINES FOR LOCATING INFORMATION ON THE INTERNET

More and more families are utilizing the Internet on a regular basis to research a wide range of topics. Many families have access to the Internet in their home, workplace, school, and at their local public library. If families are using the Internet to search for health information related to pregnancy issues and the baby, they may need assistance locating accurate and up-to-date information as well as evaluating the information they find.

Drake (1999) discussed that anyone can create an Internet site and that it is up to the user to determine the accuracy of the information. This can be frustrating for families as they begin to discover contradictory and conflicting information in their searches and are unsure of how to choose the most appropriate information for their situation. Ahmann (2000), Brooks (2001), and Lamp and Howard (1999) recommended that several issues be considered when health care sites on the Internet are evaluated. These include identification of the author or organization, date the information was posted or updated, accuracy of the content, and how well the site is maintained. Brooks also provided a comprehensive checklist to assist nurses in evaluating health care information found on the Internet. Families should be encouraged to discuss the information they find during their Internet searches so that the health care team can help them evaluate it.

FAMILY INTERNET RESOURCES

Locating health care information on the Internet can be time consuming. Dhillon, Albersheim, Alsaad, Pargass, and Zupancic (2003) surveyed parents who had a baby hospitalized in the NICU and reported that the majority found their information by using keywords to search rather than looking up specific sites. They also discussed that parents used the Internet less frequently during the baby's NICU hospitalization due to increased stress and less available time. Families that utilize the Internet may benefit from suggestions of specific web sites. This can help reduce the time they spend searching for information and also help them locate accurate and up-to-date information during their pregnancy and the baby's hospitalization. The information they find can supplement that provided by the baby's health care team and can be shared with other family members, such as grandparents and siblings. The following web sites are examples of some that might be shared with families. As with all information, they should be reviewed before being recommended.

Bed Rest

- Sidelines National Support Network—http://www.sidelines.org

Medical and Developmental Information

- American Academy of Pediatrics—http://www.aap.org
- Medline Plus—http://medlineplus.gov
- Nemours Foundation: *Kids Health*—http://www.kidshealth.org
- Web MD—http://www.webmd.com
- ZERO TO THREE—http://www.zerotothree.com

Multiple Births

- Australia Multiple Birth Association—http://www.amba.org.au/content/resources/hom
- Mothers of Supertwins—http://www.mostonline.org/
- Multiple Births/Naissances Multiples Canada—http://www.multiplebirthscanada.org/english/index.php
- National Organization of Mothers of Twins Clubs, Inc.—http://www.nomotc.org/
- The Triplet Connection—http://www.tripletconnection.com
- Twins and Multiple Births Association—http://www.tamba.org.uk/
- Twins Club—http://www.twinsclub.co.uk
- Twins List—http://www.twinslist.org

Prematurity

- March of Dimes: *Prematurity*—http://www.marchofdimes.com/prematurity/nicu/index.asp
- NICHD Neonatal Research Network: *Information for Families*—http://neonatal.rti.org/family/
- Parents of Premature Babies Inc.—http://www.preemie-l.org

- Premature Baby—Premature Child—http://www.prematurity.org
- University of Wisconsin Medical School, Department of Pediatrics: *For Parents of Preemies: Answers to Commonly Asked Questions*—http://www.pediatrics.wisc.edu/patientcare/preemies

Sick Newborns

- University of Wisconsin Medical School, Department of Pediatrics: *My Sick Newborn*—http://www.pediatrics.wisc.edu/patientcare/sicknewborn

Specific Diagnoses

Cleft Lip and Palate

- Cleft Palate Foundation—http://www.cleftline.org
- Wide Smiles: Cleft Lip and Palate Resources—http://www.widesmiles.org

Congenital Diaphragmatic Hernia

- CHERUBS: The Association of Congenital Diaphragmatic Hernia Research, Advocacy, and Support—http://www.cherubs-cdh.org

Congenital Heart Disease

- American Heart Association—http://www.americanheart.org
- Congenital Heart Information Network—http://tchin.org
- Heart Point: *Heart Point Gallery*—http://www.heartpoint.com/gallery.html

Down Syndrome

- National Down Syndrome Society—http://www.ndss.org

Group B Strep

- Group B Strep Association—http://www.groupbstrep.org

Hearing Loss

- Boys Town National Research Hospital: *My Baby's Hearing*—http://www.babyhearing.org

PKU

- Children's PKU Network—http://www.pkunetwork.org

RSV

- RSV Protection—http://www.rsvprotection.com

Spina Bifida

- Spina Bifida Association—http://www.sbaa.org/site/PageServer?page-name=index

Tracheostomy

- Aaron's Tracheostomy Page—http://www.tracheostomy.com

Twin to Twin Transfusion Syndrome

- Twin to Twin Transfusion Syndrome Australia Inc.—http://www.twin-twin.org

- Twin to Twin Transfusion Syndrome Foundation—http://www.tttsfoundation.org

Vision Loss

- Blind Children's Center—http://www.blindcntr.org/

- ROPARD: The Association for Retinopathy of Prematurity and Related Retinal Diseases—http://www.ropard.org

SIBLING INTERNET RESOURCES

Siblings may also need information on how to locate current and accurate information on the Internet. Some siblings may believe that everything they see in print, on television, or on the Internet is true no matter how inappropriate or far-fetched it may seem. Older school-age, preteen, and adolescent siblings usually feel comfortable using computers and enjoy surfing the Internet for information and activities. Therefore, when they have questions about the baby's issues, they may utilize the Internet as a resource for information. The following list includes web sites that siblings may find helpful, but there may be other excellent web sites worth checking as well. These resources should be reviewed for developmental appropriateness, accuracy, safety, and suitability before they are recommended to siblings and families.

Disability or Ongoing Medical Condition

- Club Brave Kids—http://bravekids.org

- Siblings Australia—http://www.siblingsaustralia.org.au

- The Sibling Support Project—http://www.thearc.org/siblingsupport

General Health Information

- BrainPOP: Health, Science, Technology, Math, English Animation and Education Site—http://www.brainpop.com

- Centers for Disease Control and Prevention: *BAM! Body and Mind*—http://www.bam.gov

- Kids Health—http://www.kidshealth.org/kid/

- MEDtropolis Virtual Body—http://www.medtropolis.com/VBody.aspx

Grief

- The Compassionate Friends Inc.—http://www.compassionatefriends.org

- Kids Aid—http://www.kidsaid.org

Specific Diagnoses

Congenital Diaphragmatic Hernia

- CHERUBS: The Association of Congenital Diaphragmatic Hernia Research, Advocacy, and Support—http://www.cherubs-cdh.org

Lissencephaly

- Lissencephaly Network Inc.—http://www.lissencephaly.org

ON-LINE SAFETY INFORMATION

If information is shared with families about on-line resources for siblings, information about on-line safety should be shared as well. Some parents may be aware of safety issues but are too stressed or exhausted to be as attentive as they have in the past. Also, due to the mother's hospitalization or parents' visits to the NICU, siblings may be supervised by caregivers who know little about Internet safety. Safety information can be especially important in families where the children know more about computers and the Internet than their parents do because parents may underestimate the possible dangers. Siblings may also be the family member designated to look up information on suggested web sites, as well as search for additional information about the baby's diagnosis. The following sites provide information about on-line safety for children and teens, but each site should be reviewed to ensure that it is appropriate for a particular family.

- American Academy of Child and Adolescent Psychiatry: *Children Online*—http://www.aacap.org/publications/factsfam/online.htm

- American Academy of Pediatrics: *The Internet and Your Family*—http://www.aap.org/family/interfamily.htm

- Federal Bureau of Investigation: *Safety Tips: Internet Safety*—http://www.fbi.gov/kids/k5th/safety2.htm

- Federal Trade Commission: *Kidz Privacy: Just for Kids*—http://www.ftc.gov/bcp/conline/edcams/kidzprivacy/kidz.htm

- Federal Trade Commission: *Kidz Privacy: Adults Only*—http://ftc.gov/bcp/conline/edcams/kidzprivacy/adults.htm

- Girls Health: *Safety—How to be Safety Savvy*—http://www.girlshealth.gov/safety/internet.htm

- KidsHealth: *Safe Cyberspace Surfing*—http://www.kidshealth.org/kid/watch/house/internet_safety.html

- KidsHealth: *Internet Safety*—http://www.kidshealth.org/parent/postive/family/net_safety.html

- Microsoft: *A Parent's Guide to Online Safety: Ages and Stages*—http://www.microsoft.com/athome/security/children/parentsguide.mspx

- Netsmartz: *Internet Safety Pledges*—http://www.netsmartz.org/resources/pledge.htm

BOOKS FOR SIBLINGS

Reading books together can help family members cope with various aspects of pregnancy, the baby's hospitalization, or the baby's death. Families can benefit from recommendations of specific books as well as locations to find appropriate books. The following list should serve only as a guide because there are other excellent publications available that can be found at local bookstores, libraries, and on-line. In the following list, resources supplied by a particular company are accompanied by a web site. As with any resource, all of the books in this list should be reviewed before being shared with families.

Hospitalization of the Baby

- Duncan, D. (1994). *When Molly was in the hospital: A book for brothers and sisters of hospitalized children.* Windsor, CA: Rayve Productions.

- Klayman, G.J. (2001). *Our new baby needs special help: A coloring workbook for families whose new baby has problems* (Revised ed.). Omaha, NE: Centering Corp.; http://www.centering.org

- Jaworski, A.M., & Ball, L. (1998). *My brother needs an operation.* Temple, TX: Baby Hearts Press.

Death and Dying Issues

- Al-Chokhachy, E. (1998). *The angel with the golden glow.* Marblehead, MA: Penny Bear.

- Cohn, J. (1994). *Molly's rosebush.* Morton Grove, IL: Albert Whitman & Co.

- Grollman, E., & Johnson, J. (2001). *A child's book about death.* Omaha, NE: Centering Corp.; http://www.centering.org

- Gryte, M. (1999). *No new baby.* Omaha, NE: Centering Corp.; http://www.centering.org

- Johnson, J., & Johnson, M. (1982). *Where's Jess?* Omaha, NE: Centering Corp.; http://www.centering.org

- Johnson, P.P. (1993). *Morgan's baby sister: A read-aloud book for families who have experienced the death of a newborn.* San Jose, CA: Resource Publications.

- Keough, P. (2001). *Remembering our baby: A workbook for children whose brother or sister dies before birth.* Omaha, NE: Centering Corp.; http://www.centering.org

- *My always sister coloring book.* (n.d.). St. Paul, MN: A Place to Remember; http://www.aplacetoremember.com

- Old, W.C. (1995). *Stacy had a little sister.* Morton Grove, IL: Albert Whitman & Co.

- Parkinson, S. (1995). *All shining in the spring: The story of a baby who died.* Dublin, Ireland: O'Brien Press.

- Schwiebert, P. (2003). *We were gonna have a baby, but we had an angel instead.* Portland, OR: Grief Watch; http://www.griefwatch.com

- Simon, J., & Simon, A. (2002). *This book is for all kids, but especially my sister Libby. Libby died.* Kansas City, MO: Andrews McMeel Publishing.

- Tapp, K.K. (1998). *No smile cookies today.* Wayzata, MN: Pregnancy and Infant Loss Center; http://www.nationalshareoffice.com

Maternal Bed Rest

- *My mommy is on bed rest coloring book.* (n.d.). St. Paul, MN: A Place to Remember; http://www.aplacetoremember.com

- Travis, H.M. (1999). *And mommy's on her side.* St. Paul, MN: A Place to Remember; http://www.aplacetoremember.com

Multiple Births

- Bergren, L.T. (2001). *God gave us two*. Colorado Springs, CO: Water-Brook Press.

- Bunting, E. (1997). *Twinnies*. San Diego: Harcourt Brace & Co.

- Dewan, T. (2003). *Crispin and the 3 little piglets*. New York: Random House.

- Snyder, C. (1995). *One up, one down*. New York: Atheneum.

Prematurity

- Amadeo, D.M. (2005). *My baby sister is a preemie*. Grand Rapids, MI: Zonder Kids.

- Collins, P.L. (1990). *Waiting for baby Joe*. Niles, IL: Albert Whitman & Co.

- Hawkins-Walsh, E. (2002). *Katie's premature brother* (Revised ed.). Omaha, NE: Centering Corp.; http://www.centering.org

- Lafferty, L., & Flood, B. (1998). *Born early: A premature baby's story*. Minneapolis, MN: Fairview Press.

- *My preemie brother coloring book*. (n.d.). St. Paul, MN: A Place to Remember; http://www.aplacetoremember.com

- Murphy-Melas, E. (1996). *Watching Bradley grow: A story about premature birth*. Georgia: Longstreet Press.

- Pankow, V. (2004). *No bigger than my teddy bear* (Revised ed.). Petaluma, CA: Family Books; http://www.preemie.com

- Resta, B. (1995). *Believe in Katie Lynn*. Nashville: Eggman.

- Wild, M., & Brooks, R. (1999). *Rosie and Tortoise*. New York: DK Publishing.

- Wilkie, D. (1990). *Mommy, what is a preemie?* Minneapolis, MN: International Childbirth Education Association; http://www.preemie.com

Sibling and Coping Issues

- Cutler, J. (1993). *Darcy and Gran don't like babies*. New York: Scholastic.

- Danziger, P. (2004). *Barfburger baby, I was here first*. New York: G.P. Putnam's Sons.

- Douglas, A. (1998). *Baby science*. Toronto: Owl Books.

- Ellis, S. (2005). *That baby woke me up, again*. Charleston, SC: BookSurge.

- Fisher, V. (2002). *My big brother*. New York: Atheneum Books for Young Readers.

- Fisher, V. (2003). *My big sister.* New York: Atheneum Books for Young Readers.

- Henkes, K. (1990). *Julius, the baby of the world.* New York: Greenwillow Books.

- Hiatt, F. (1999). *Baby talk.* New York: Simon & Schuster.

- Mario, H.S. (1999). *I'd rather have an iguana.* Watertown, MA: Charlesbridge.

- Michels-Gualtieri, A.S. (2003). *I was born to be a sister.* Washington, DC: Platypus Media.

- Michels-Gualtieri, Z.G. (2003). *I was born to be a brother.* Washington, DC: Platypus Media.

- Palatini, M. (2000). *Good as Goldie.* New York: Hyperion.

- Penn, A. (2004). *A pocket full of kisses.* Washington, DC: Child & Family Press.

- Ross, T. (2000). *Wash your hands!* La Jolla, CA: Kane/Miller.

- Sheldon, A. (2006). *Big sister: Now a story about me and our new baby.* Washington, DC: Magination Press.

- Sullivan, S. (2005). *Dear baby letters from your big brother.* Cambridge, MA: Candlewick Press.

- Wahl, J. (2000). *Mabel ran away with the toys.* Watertown, MA: Charlesbridge.

- Whybrow, I. (2001). *A baby for Grace.* Boston: Houghton Mifflin.

- Winter, S. (1994). *A baby just like me.* New York: DK Children.

Specific Diagnoses

- Lowell, G.R. (2000). *Elana's ears or how I became the best big sister in the world.* Washington, DC: Magination Press.

- Metzger, L. (1992). *Barry's sister.* New York: Macmillan.

- Peckinpah, S.L. (1991). *Rosey, the imperfect angel.* Woodline Hills, CA: Scholars Press.

- Rheingrover, J.S. (1996). *Veronica's first year.* Morton Grove, IL: Albert Whitman & Co.

- Stuve-Bodeen, S. (1998). *We'll paint the octopus red.* Bethesda, MD: Red Woodbine House.

Stepfamily Issues

- Ballard, R. (1998). *When I am a sister.* New York: Greenwillow Books.

Index

Page numbers followed by *f* indicate figures; those followed by *t* indicate tables.

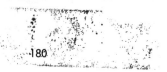